TEEN PREGNANCY CHALLENGE

Book Two

Also by Jeanne Lindsay and Sharon Rodine:

Teen Pregnancy Challenge, Book One: Strategies for Change

By Jeanne Lindsay and Catherine Monserrat:

*Adoption Awareness: Help for Teachers,
Counselors, Nurses and Caring Others*

By Jeanne Warren Lindsay:

*Teens Parenting: The Challenge of Babies and Toddlers
Do I Have a Daddy? A Story About a Single-Parent Child
Teenage Marriage: Coping with Reality
Teens Look at Marriage: Rainbows, Roles and Reality
Parents, Pregnant Teens and the Adoption Option:
Help for Families
Pregnant Too Soon: Adoption Is an Option
Open Adoption: A Caring Option*

TEEN PREGNANCY CHALLENGE

Book Two
Programs for Kids

Jeanne Warren Lindsay, M.A., C.H.E.

and

Sharon Rodine, M.Ed.

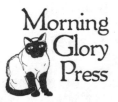

Morning
Glory
Press

Buena Park, California

Library of Congress Cataloging-in-Publication Data

Lindsay, Jeanne Warren.
    Teen pregnancy challenge.

    Includes bibliographical references.
    Contents: v. 1. Strategies for change --
v. 2. Programs for kids.
    1. Teenage mothers--United States. 2. Teenage pregnancy--
United States. 3. Social work with teenagers--United States.
I. Rodine, Sharon.   II. Title.
    HQ759.4.L559 1989   362.7'96   89-14491
    ISBN 0-930934-41-5 (set)
    ISBN 0-930934-40-7 (set : pbk.)
    ISBN 0-930934-35-0 (v. 1)
    ISBN 0-930934-34-2 (v. 1 : pbk.)
    ISBN 0-930934-39-3 (v. 2)
    ISBN 0-930934-38-5 (v. 2 : pbk.)

MORNING GLORY PRESS, INC.
6595 San Haroldo Way   Buena Park, CA 90620
Telephone (714) 828-1998
Printed and bound in the United States of America

*To caring people everywhere
who work at some point
on the adolescent pregnancy prevention continuum
to make life a little better
for our young people.*

Morning Glory Press, Inc.
is pleased to publish

Teen Pregnancy Challenge, Book One and *Book Two*

in cooperation with

The National Organization on Adolescent Pregnancy
and Parenting, Inc. (NOAPP)

NOAPP is a national membership network dedicated
to preventing adolescent pregnancy
and problems related to adolescent sexuality,
pregnancy and parenting.

To join NOAPP, or for information, contact
Executive Director
NOAPP
P.O. Box 2365
Reston, VA 22090
703/435-3948

Contents

    Future planning may be difficult; Magical thinking
    prevails; May lack self identity; Why don't they use
    birth control? Special health services for teens; Unique
    group with unique needs.

Preface

Too-early pregnancy is a challenge to the young men and women involved. Helping young people avoid too-early pregnancy and providing assistance to those already pregnant or parenting is one of the biggest challenges facing all of us who care about young people. Whether we're speaking of emotional, social and physical damage to young parents and their children, or concentrating on the economic costs to society brought about by too-early pregnancy, prevention is the best antidote.

Included in this prevention package is prevention of too-early sexual involvement among our youth, prevention of pregnancy for young people already sexually active, prevention of health and psychosocial problems among pregnant teenagers, their partners, and their babies, and help in preventing some of the many problems faced by young parents and their children.

All across the country, schools, churches, health services, and other youth-serving agencies are offering programs targeting young people all along this prevention continuum. Any of us planning to start or expand teen pregnancy prevention or care services profit the most from visiting successful programs with goals similar to our own, and in listening to the people behind these programs.

Teen Pregnancy Challenge, Book Two: Programs for Kids cannot transport you to Arizona, Florida, Maine, Oklahoma, or California to visit successful programs, but it does give you an opportunity to learn from and about programs in these and many other states. And if, after reading about these programs, you would like a person-to-person conversation, you are encouraged to contact program personnel through the resource listing in the Appendix.

There are many excellent adolescent pregnancy prevention and care programs in the United States. Those included in this book present examples of various types of approaches being used in local communities, both large and small. This book is meant to give you ideas, to stimulate your thinking, and to help you consider the range of innovative program possibilities that could be initiated in your home community. Our wish is that, while reading this book, you will say, "We could do that right here!"

Foreword

All of us in the field of sexual and reproductive health continually comment that young people who live in risky environments need to be cared for and provided for in a special way. Essentially, we are saying that our children are our future. They need us to show them the way to independence, self sufficiency, and the development of feelings of self-esteem and self-worth. This book provides important insights and directions about how these outcomes can be achieved programmatically in community agencies, institutions, and schools.

Jeanne Lindsay and Sharon Rodine have carefully put together a solid book which centers on very concrete approaches to working with teens and families in a variety of settings. A recurring emphasis throughout this valuable work is the critical nature of the problem of unintended pregnancy and childbearing in the teen years. Their message is clear. The prospects for teen parents and their children for a healthy and independent life are significantly reduced.

Young mothers are at an enormous risk of pregnancy complications and poor birth outcomes, and their infants face great health and developmental risks. Teenage parents are more likely than those who delay childbearing to experience chronic unemployment, inadequate income, reduced educational experiences, and the burden of feelings of relentless fatalism. They and their children are very likely to become dependent on public assistance and to remain dependent for a long period of time. The emotional toll on these young people is staggering and incalculable.

Society's economic burden in sustaining families that begin with the birth of a child to a teen is now running close to twenty billion dollars a year.

We have already learned that the beginning of wisdom in dealing realistically with this national health concern is the recognition of the stark reality of the teenage pregnancy and childbearing situation. It is a situation that has been facing us for some time now, and has been long in developing. It has been, and continues to be, conditioned by many complex racial, economic, educational, family, and other social factors.

Clearly, adolescent pregnancy in America is a complex situation, and therefore, requires complex interventions. There are no quick fix solutions; no single intervention programs that will do the job; no slick button phrases or bumper stickers which by themselves will reduce the haunting, unacceptable statistics, and their impact in human terms on the lives of so many young people. The authors point out that individuals, community agencies, and schools must endeavor to meet this challenge with new enthusiasm and renewed resolve.

What is very clear from the program descriptions presented by Lindsay and Rodine is that the way to deal with this problem is not simply to help our young people develop the capacity to avoid unintended pregnancy and to develop the cognitive abilities required to make responsible sexual decisions. At the same time we are trying to achieve these important outcomes, we must provide our youth with opportunities for life-change possibilities that will yield within them a desire not to become pregnant at this time in their development. It is clearly pointed out that young people need to be provided better pathways to concrete, meaningful, and fulfilling options in their lives. What is also clear in *Programs for Kids* is the importance of devising multi-dimensional, holistic approaches with both teen females and teen males that help develop within them a positive sense and value of themselves, a range of life-coping skills, and the ability to be appropriately assertive about their needs and concerns.

Conversely, without this help, many teen females and males do not see a future for themselves. They see poor employment opportunities around them, and face the prospect of life-long poor economic status and inadequate opportunity for meaningful education. The specter of hopelessness about their possibility for success in life becomes vivid and daunting. Under such conditions it is clear that some young people choose to become sexually irresponsible and fatalistic instead of becoming sexually responsible, industrious, and hopeful.

Much of what is contained in this valuable book provides insight, guidance, and practical tools for creating an upbeat and positive climate for young people who are in need of our support and affection. In particular, the section on working with teen males is especially stimulating and useful. The programs described provide essential information on approaches for working with teen males that are at once attractive, focused, and engaging. The emphases in these descriptions are right on target. That is, the way toward achieving male responsibility in sexual expression is through success in careers and employment, and through achievement in academics, (both of which produce enhanced self-esteem), as well as through knowledge of contraception.

In addition, the chapters on services and programs for pregnant teens and teens who have had a child are extremely valuable. They communicate the need to provide support to young people and families who continue to need comprehensive services while we in the field continue to rework our primary prevention approaches.

I feel this book is among the most practical and useful treatments of this critical issue. I know it will create a new national awareness to the challenge that is facing us in our work with young people and will stimulate more assertive and creative programming. Needy teens and families throughout the country are the beneficiaries of this important book.

Michael Carrera
Thomas Hunter Professor of Health Sciences
Hunter College, New York
Director, Dunlevy-Milbank Teenage Pregnancy Prevention
    Program, New York City

Acknowledgments

In *Teen Pregnancy Challenge, Book One: Strategies for Change,* we acknowledged the many people who helped us with these books. We again express our deep gratitude to these wonderful individuals.

We interviewed in depth at least one hundred people and talked with many, many more. Some of them sent lovely photographs of the young people in their programs, and we included several in each volume of *Teen Pregnancy Challenge.* We regret that we could not use all of them.

People who are quoted in this volume or whose programs are described are listed in the Appendix, pages 217-226. An apt title for this section would be "Acknowledgments, Part Two." We appreciate so much the help these people provided.

Ellen Peach, Mary Ann Liebert, Barbara Huberman, Sue Dolezal, Caroline Gaston, Marie E. Mitchell, Lois Gatchell, Genie Wheeler, Erin B. Lindsay, and Dick Rodine critiqued the *Book Two* manuscript.

All the NOAPP Board members have been supportive as always.

Betty Dodson, co-founder and former director of the El Paso, Texas, Project Redirection, wrote a history of that program and sent it to us because, she said, "It's too complicated to describe verbally." We were intrigued with the wide variety and the comprehensiveness of the services provided by Project Redirection, so much so that, with Betty's permission, we included it in *Teen Pregnancy Challenge, Book One*. We consider it an inspiration for the rest of us as we design programs to help young people. We appreciate Betty's contribution to *Teen Pregnancy Challenge*.

Carole Blum proof-read tirelessly—in the office, at home, and on the freeway (she wasn't driving). We hereby proclaim her an MP—Master Proofreader.

Michael and Brent Rodine have been tolerant as their mother worked through the many drafts of these chapters.

The Lindsay kids are grown and gone, but Eric, Pati, and Mike continue to encourage by phone, while Erin and Steve are involved in editing and book design, respectively.

Our spouses, Dick Rodine and Bob Lindsay, continue to be supportive, loving, and caring, although we suspect both are even more delighted than we are that these books are completed.

We have appreciated each other's patience, and we've enjoyed working together.

Jeanne Lindsay
Sharon Rodine

Introduction

Some people use the phrase "adolescent pregnancy prevention continuum" to refer only to programs ranging from primary prevention (saying "No" to too-early sexual intercourse) through preventing too-early pregnancy among teenagers already sexually active. However, the continuum goes on to include programs providing for healthy pregnancies and healthy babies through early prenatal care for pregnant teens, and programs offering support services for teenage parents and their children.

The National Organization on Adolescent Pregnancy and Parenting, Inc. (NOAPP) is a membership organization of service providers and community leaders at the local and state level who work diligently to prevent too-early childbearing, and to provide needed services for pregnant and parenting teens.

As NOAPP's executive director (Sharon Rodine) and newsletter editor (Jeanne Lindsay), we have collected information on hundreds of adolescent pregnancy programs providing prevention or care intervention services at the local community level. We interviewed in depth many people involved in providing these services, and talked with and/or received written information from several hundred others.

We could not include all the agencies and programs we contacted in gathering information for these books. A vast amount of additional care and prevention program information is included in NOAPP's resource files, available on request.

Many states have statewide organizations addressing teen pregnancy issues. In others, key agencies and individuals have been identified. Names, addresses, and phone numbers of these state contacts are listed in the Appendix of this volume.

Originally, this book was simply an extra section in *Teen Pregnancy Challenge: Strategies for Change*. We planned to describe a few programs along the teen pregnancy prevention continuum as examples of the diversity of programs helping young people. We already had written descriptions, usually fairly brief, of programs coordinated by many members of NOAPP. We wrote a few descriptions from this information, but realized we wanted more details. So we started interviewing.

As we talked with program directors across the country, we became more and more excited by the enthusiasm and the caring for kids these people demonstrated. It was similar to conference encounters, where we meet new people in our field and are enthralled with the insight these conversations bring.

About midway through the book-writing process, we realized we had outgrown our one-book concept. We were doing two things at once. We were writing a book on developing programs, as we had planned. We were deeply into discussions of documenting the need, gaining community support, planning content and setting, raising money, the evaluation process, and other aspects of program development.

All of these topics were relevant for program development at any point on the adolescent pregnancy prevention continuum. Whether the program is designed to help preschoolers gain a sense of self-esteem, middle school children learn the assertive skills needed for saying "No" to too-early sexual involvement, sexually active youth delay pregnancy until they are ready to parent, or provide services for pregnant and parenting teenagers and their children, these tasks are necessary for the development of a successful program.

But we also wanted to be more specific about programs at different points on that continuum. As we talked with the service providers, we decided this second book was an important part of our *Teen Pregnancy Challenge.* We realized we wanted to "listen" to people talk about their programs at their chosen spot on that continuum. For many, the "chosen spot" is itself a continuum. So often as we talked with people running programs for teen parents, for example, we learned they, too, were involved in pregnancy prevention programs.

Over and over we heard, "Prevention is the answer. Intervention after the fact of pregnancy is necessary, but preventing the pregnancy is the economical intervention, economical in human and financial terms."

We must provide care for teen parents and their children— without intervention services, the costs of allowing those young families to flounder in poverty and despair are simply too high. At the same time, prevention of too-early pregnancy must have high priority.

This is not a catalog of programs. Selected features of selected programs are described to demonstrate the possibilities for helping young people. Selection of programs to be featured was somewhat arbitrary. We aren't suggesting that these are the only, or even the best programs for the needs addressed. Each, however, appears to have a strong foundation of caring concern for young people, an overriding conviction that intervention is needed, and that the right intervention can improve the lives of our young people.

Deciding who to interview was a frustrating task. We wanted to focus on programs currently active. Some are quite unique while others represent a number of similar offerings. We knew the impossibility of choosing the best programs throughout the United States because that would clearly be a subjective decision. It is not necessary or even appropriate to believe programs should be rated in that manner.

Our goal was to talk in depth with directors of a wide variety of programs, directors with experience in health services or in the schools or churches or social services, people who work with teenagers and people who work with preschoolers and their parents. We wanted to let the reader hear from people representing the tremendous variety of services that are available, and to hear from families and their communities. If we truly expect to make a dent in the wall of problems surrounding the phenomenon of too-early pregnancy, we must share the wealth of information already available. We don't need to reinvent the wheel; instead, we can continue to build on successes that have already been achieved.

The people quoted are performing these services with widely varying approaches to the teen pregnancy challenge. We salute them all—and we salute the others, those we didn't interview but who are out there helping kids, their families, and their communities deal with the challenge of too-early pregnancy and parenting.

No matter which age group you decide you want to target— preschoolers and their families, pre-adolescents, or adolescents—what can you and your community do to help those children and young people develop high self-esteem and the ability and drive to achieve their goals? This, of course, is the best possible antidote to too-early pregnancy.

As we emphasize in this book and in its companion, *Teen Pregnancy Challenge, Book 1: Strategies for Change*, some young people from all socio-economic levels, all ethnic groups, and all kinds of families get pregnant before the rest of the world thinks they're ready. However, those living in poverty, those who have dropped out of school, have no job skills, and very little hope of leading productive lives, are most likely to become pregnant too soon. Abstinence and contraception are important parts of postponing pregnancy. Self-esteem and an achievable plan for a promising future are an integral part of the same script.

Each of us, whoever and wherever we are, can help young people. Identify your spot on the intervention continuum, and begin to develop programs needed to meet the *Teen Pregnancy Challenge* in your community.

CHAPTER 1

Understanding Adolescence

Adolescence is a complicated developmental phase. As their bodies change drastically, young people are trying to figure out who they are, trying to shape their adult identities. For many youth, this is a time of rebellion, a time when much of what they have been taught, what they have believed, is suddenly challenged. It is a time when teens test their independence.

Many teenagers resent being told what to do. Peer pressure is likely to have more effect on their behavior than parental directives. Many are highly resistant to what they term "preaching." Helping them learn to make healthy choices themselves is likely to produce better results over time than are too many "No, you can'ts."

Adults tend to see teenagers themselves as the problem while it may be more realistic to think of the world around them as the problem. Perhaps then, it is possible to understand that our role is to help adolescents through this period of transition from childhood to maturity, rather than making life even more

difficult for them. Parents and others working with adolescents
need to remember that normal behavior during adolescence
often involves pushing the rules and challenging authority.

This stage is also hard on the adolescent's parents because no
longer can they "make everything right" for their children. We
have to let teens make choices and face the consequences, and
that's difficult for parents.

Communication between parents and their children is extremely important during the teen years. Good communication
develops over time, and ideally starts in early childhood. Waiting until the teen years is too late to start open communication.

Young people find puberty confusing. They need to know
why their bodies are changing, and this knowledge can help
them feel good about themselves. "Just say '*KNOW*'—teens
need to **KNOW**" is a good approach. Understanding themselves
helps them cope with the stresses of adolescence. *Not* knowing
the changes taking place within themselves, both physically and
psychologically, is the dangerous approach.

Future Planning May Be Difficult

Teenagers tend to live for the moment. For many, their
developmental stage doesn't yet allow much serious planning
for the future. Adolescents may still be in the concrete stage of
thinking, and actually be unable cognitively to plan far into the
future.

She's in love today and this is forever. He thinks having a
baby would make him a man, and he doesn't think about the
eighteen years of fatherhood he could be facing. The future isn't
a career with a pension; it's the dance tomorrow night.

Ellen Peach, co-author of **Family TALKS,** has worked with
many adolescents. When asked, "How do you work with a
fourteen-year-old?" she replied:

> *Everything is today, **now.** If it has no relevance to
> where she is today, it has no relevance at all. You can't
> even go to next week. If she's pregnant and you want to
> talk about cigarette smoking, you have to talk about where
> the baby is now and where she is now.*

> *If she's able to look ahead, you can pick that up*
> *through her comments. If she says something about*
> *money, that indicates to me that she can look ahead, that*
> *she's thinking in terms of consequences. She may be ready*
> *to deal with hypothetical thinking.*

Many teens live only for the here and now. They also feel invincible. "Of course I can drink and drive. I can handle it." "It won't happen to me." If we're honest, most of us can remember our own risk-taking behavior when we were adolescents. Besides, adult society promotes the risk-taking, go-for-it attitudes.

Teens in a recent survey showed little concern about dealing with unplanned pregnancy. Only sixteen percent listed this as a top concern. Yet only eighteen percent of the surveyed teens "believe teen parenthood is all right."

The survey was carried out in 1988 by the American Home Economics Association with funding from Chesebrough-Pond's, Inc., and Lever Brothers Company. It was designed to answer questions about how teenagers view themselves and the world around them (*Journal of Home Economics*, Summer, 1989, pages 27-40).

We know that teens who do well academically are less likely to get pregnant, or to cause a pregnancy too soon, than are teens who are failing their classes. However, convincing a teen that studying today will make a difference in her/his earning power ten years from now is difficult. They are likely to want concrete results *now*, and getting good grades may not be reward enough for some young people.

Beth Brandes was concerned that the majority of the young women in the **Teen Talk Program, Forsyth County, North Carolina,** were underachieving at school. She asked them, "What would it take to improve your grades?"

"Ten dollars," they replied.

Someone had donated $250 to the program, so Brandes decided to accommodate her clients. Anyone who had a certain grade in every class at the end of the semester was paid $10. The first time this incentive was offered, eight of the teenagers

NO FUN.

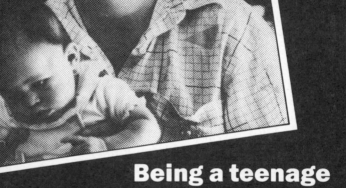

**Being a teenage parent.
It's 24 hours a day.**

Every day.

PARENTS *Too Soon*

**HOTLINE:
1·800·4·CALL US**

A Program of the State of Illinois

earned the "incentive compensation," and the next time, fourteen did. After-school tutoring was an important part of the program.

Brandes talked about the criticism sometimes directed at this kind of reward system, and of how she used the situation to generate positive interest in the program:

> *People say, "I don't believe in paying for grades."*
> *I say, "I understand that, but my guess is that you reward your children in different ways. You take your child out for pizza," or you say, "When you're eighteen you can have a car." These kids don't have that.*
>
> *We were able to generate other revenue because the academic achievement program was a saleable thing. Dropout prevention and academic achievement are so much more acceptable than sexuality. A lot of people will buy into that who would never dream of backing sexuality education.*
>
> *I think we have to have vision about how we will present this program to the public. I don't make any bones about presenting sexuality education, but you can't just talk about a kid's uterus. You have to talk about the other things you're accomplishing, the kids whose grades improve, who get jobs, who start making healthy decisions. At that point, people want to help.*

Magical Thinking Prevails

The "It can't happen to me" outlook often carries over into thinking about contraception and pregnancy. Anyone working with pregnant adolescents has heard, "But I didn't think I'd get pregnant," or "I hope I'm not."

The magical thinking of adolescence makes it difficult to help them make responsible decisions concerning their sexuality.

This magical thinking may cause a pregnant teen to tell no one about her pregnancy, almost as if she doesn't believe it's happening. "If I don't talk about it, maybe it'll go away." A challenge for parents and other helping persons is to provide an environment in which sexual issues may be discussed openly.

Adolescents are absolutely sure everyone is watching them. They worry about how they look, and about their perceived lack of popularity. They are extremely sensitive to criticism, and their self-esteem is easily damaged.

Neither partner can talk to the other about contraception or about AIDS because "I'd be too embarrassed." Teenagers' failure to use health clinic services may stem from embarrassment or fear that others will know what they're doing. They may not have enough information about the services to feel comfortable using them.

Embarrassment may keep a young person from discussing sexual issues with his/her parents. And parents may feel the same kind of embarrassment in spite of their personal distance from their own adolescence.

As the teenager searches for her own identity, she is also continuing to develop her own value system. That value system may not condone premarital sex. It would be wrong, she feels, to plan to have sexual intercourse before marriage. To be contraceptively prepared, therefore, is wrong. But if she is "swept away" by the passion of the moment, it's okay and she can't be blamed. The result is likely to be an unplanned—but very real—pregnancy.

Most helping persons applaud adolescents' attempts to make decisions based on their own value systems. We're pleased if that value system supports a young person's decision not to have premarital intercourse. In addition, however, we must help that young person develop the skills she (or he) will need to stick with that value system. The "Just say 'No'" technique may not be strong enough to withstand peer pressure. Assertiveness training, along with life skills and goal setting, is more effective.

May Lack Self Identity

Self-esteem and self-confidence play important roles in teen sexual behavior. A teen with low self-confidence may not be able to say "No" to a boyfriend or girlfriend. She may become sexually active because this makes her feel somebody likes her. If she says "No," she may lose her boyfriend. If he doesn't push sex, he's afraid his girlfriend will find someone who will.

A teen girl who has not yet found her own identity may cling to her boyfriend, feeling her sense of worth comes from being with him. Her boyfriend may have the same problem. Sometimes we see couples who appear to be so dependent on each other that neither is able to develop the self-identity so important in a strong relationship.

Heather, a fourteen-year-old mother, shared with her teacher that she had finally broken up with her sometimes abusive boyfriend. The teacher commented on the courage such a decision requires.

"Oh, it's all right," Heather responded. "I have a new boyfriend—and just in time." In other words, Heather felt she couldn't cope by herself, apparently feeling she was "nobody" without a boyfriend.

Sara, fifteen when she realized she was pregnant, epitomizes the adolescent stage of development:

> *I was really afraid. You don't think it will happen to you. When you think of people who are pregnant, they're married, and getting pregnant just wasn't on my mind. I think I was in shock and not believing it until Benny was a week old.*
>
> *Even now I can barely remember the first year because I was so out of it.*

Sara's school apparently believed teenagers were abstinent at least until eleventh grade. She commented:

> *When I got pregnant, I was ignorant about birth control because my school didn't teach birth control until eleventh grade. We had the health classes where they teach you what happens when you get pregnant, but they never talked about how to prevent it. I guess they thought we already knew about that.*

Sara liked high school and partying with her friends. When she was fifteen she dated a twenty-year-old, and soon learned she was pregnant:

My friends called me names and spread it around the school. They wrote "Prego Bitch" on my locker, and it was real hard.

I wanted to get an abortion, but I couldn't get the money together. Telling my mom was the last thing I wanted to do, but finally she noticed it. She wasn't mad, but she was sad that I couldn't tell her. She accepted it pretty well.

I transferred to the Teen Parent Program for my sophomore year, but had to go back to the regular high school the next year, and that was awful. I got my first two Fs—failed that whole semester. The Teen Parent Program had moved to the regular high school, so I took one class there and the rest were regular classes. But I didn't go to school much.

"The kids are here and we love them,
of course, but it's rocky."

I couldn't get the pills because my cholesterol was high. I had an IUD but my mom didn't like it, so I had it taken out. So I got pregnant again. Benny was three when Jenny was born.

Finally last semester I got my act together, and my counselor thinks she can get a scholarship to an art institute for me. I hope to go straight to college after I graduate next January.

I'm living on my own with my boyfriend now. It's a little rocky—we have a hard time getting along. The kids are here and we love them, of course, but it's rocky. He's twenty-five and he's working. We've been together on and off since I got pregnant the first time.

Sometimes I go back to live with my mom, but she's an alcoholic, and she always fights with me. That's not good for the kids so I try to stay out.

The father and I lived with her for a year after Benny was born. Then she got more bossy, and it got harder to live with her.

You don't expect all the expenses you're going to have
when you first move out. That's hard even when you don't
have a kid. We've been in and out of apartments so much
because financially we can't do it. Emotionally it's
hard, too.

Why Don't They Use Birth Control?

Why do so many teens ignore birth control, yet are sexually active? Some teenagers report never using contraceptives, and about forty percent report they use them "sometimes." Many teenagers fail to use any kind of contraception the first time they have intercourse. The average delay between first intercourse and first use of a prescription method is about one year (*Risking the Future,* page 49. 1987: National Academy of Sciences).

Some teens don't know about birth control, or they may not know how to get it. Some don't know how to use contraceptives, others are too embarrassed to do so. Even buying condoms at the store may prove too embarrassing for many. As we've said before, some believe if you plan ahead, you have already made the decision to have sex. If you get swept away in the passion of the moment, then you really aren't to blame.

Some young women take the pill for a month or two, then stop. A clinic counselor reports having patients coming in for a pregnancy check when she knows they were taking the birth control pill earlier. "Why did you stop taking the pill?" she asks.

The classic answer, the one most often heard, is, "I didn't think I'd get pregnant." The clinic counselor also hears, "Somebody said I'd get fat" or "A friend said they had sugar in them." Someone may have said the pill causes cancer or heart attacks. Other teens can't afford to have the prescription refilled.

Pregnant teens may describe pregnancy as an accident. *Adults need to help young people understand that pregnancy is not an accident.*

Special Health Services for Teens

Program providers and others in the community may question the need for special services for teenagers. If the community has a health clinic, why consider adding a special

clinic for adolescents? If prenatal care services are available
for pregnant women generally, why is it even better to have
additional services provided specifically for pregnant teens?

Teens, with their tendency to live for the moment, often
need extra encouragement to obtain preventive health care.
Embarrassment may keep them out of clinics they perceive as
existing for adults. They may find the white-coated medical
staff intimidating. Services planned especially for teens are
more likely to succeed in meeting adolescents' unique
health needs.

The pregnancy and live birth rate in **Ypsilanti, Michigan**,
was double the national average, and the infant mortality rate
was high in the late seventies, according to Joan Chesler,
Executive Director, **The Corner Health Center.** Teenagers had
serious health problems, but the only health services were eight
miles away in Ann Arbor, an extremely different community.
People either went there for health care, or they didn't get any. If
they did go to Ann Arbor, it tended to be on a crisis basis. For
many families, prevention is a whole new concept, Chesler
explained.

Kids found it hard to understand why birth control was a
good idea from a preventive standpoint. Prenatal patients missed
appointments because they didn't feel sick. "The Corner Health
Center opened here because we needed to change our clients'
approach to the health care system," Chesler explained. "They
may have grown up in families where professionals are mis-
trusted, and you only see one when you absolutely have to. We
wanted to be a bridge between the physician and the mother who
is taking her baby to the doctor."

Chesler described the different approach they take to prenatal
health care for teens compared to care for adults:

> *First, we make our appointments twenty to thirty
> minutes apart. An exam takes the same amount of time
> here as in the adult care system, but the education takes
> five times as long.*
> *We spend a great deal of time helping our patients feel
> at ease as well as in describing the medical condition. We*

*explain how to treat it, then ask the patient to repeat this
back to us.*

*Our pregnant teenagers have appointments every two
weeks rather than once a month. We do this for several
reasons. First, we feel they need more medical monitoring
and observation. They need more attention, more help
with nutrition. Second, if they miss an appointment, they
expect to have to come back in two weeks—and it works.
You know, "My car broke down," "My ride didn't show
up," "I had to stay after school." Whatever the reason,
they're back two weeks later. They also come in early in
their pregnancies because we do pregnancy diagnosis and
family planning.*

*On the average, our teenage patients end up having
more than the recommended number of prenatal visits.
The minimum standard is nine, while our patients average
twelve. Our twice-monthly schedule helps us reach that.*

*We're different from adult clinics in other ways, too.
We set the radio to a soft rock station. Our clinicians are
mostly on a first-name basis with our clients. They wear
street clothes, not white coats. They look like real people
and they act like real people. We change our posters
regularly to make it look interesting. Our bathroom has a
basketful of condoms. We found that when we asked kids
to ask for condoms, they didn't.*

*Kids who would not ordinarily get any prenatal or
family planning care, the street kids, trust us enough to
come here even when they're having major difficulties in
other parts of their lives.*

Male involvement is difficult to achieve in a clinic seen
primarily as a woman's place, according to Chesler. The staff
has been reaching out more to the schools, and the outreach
groups include some teen fathers.

Chesler reports that, compared to prenatal care in a teaching
hospital, cost of prenatal care in the adolescent clinic is fifty-
nine percent less while the health outcome is the same. She
described the study done by David Share, Bonnie J. Kay, and

Kathie Jones which compared 180 prenatal health clients at The
Corner Health Center with 180 adolescent prenatal health clients
at a nearby teaching hospital. The Corner's clients made an
average of 12.8 prenatal visits while the other clients made only
9.8, a significant difference.

A higher percentage of The Corner clients either stopped or
reduced their smoking during pregnancy. Six months after
delivery, a higher percentage of The Corner clients were using
contraceptives: 78.4 percent versus 45 percent of the teaching
hospital clients. Two years after delivery, 15.4 percent of The
Corner clients were pregnant again compared to 30.4 percent of
the other group.

"We attribute these results to the more personal relationships
established in our clinic, which in turn have an impact on the
health education provided. From the health as well as from the
cost perspective, having a health center like this for kids makes a
great deal of sense," Chesler concluded.

Unique Group with Unique Needs

Adolescent men and women are a special group of people
with unique needs. As they move from childhood toward
adulthood, most need help and support as they go through this
difficult period. At the same time, many are rebelling, doing
their own thing, and appear not to want help from any of us.

Our adolescent population includes a tremendous variety of
young people. In terms of the teen pregnancy prevention continuum, individuals range from a considerable population of young
people still sexually abstinent in their mid-teens to the also
considerable population who are sexually active, some before
they reach the teen years. Teen mothers and fathers are at the
other end of the prevention continuum, young people who may
not have meant to get pregnant, but, after the fact, want to be
good parents with healthy children.

These young people, wherever they are on that continuum,
need our understanding and our help.

CHAPTER 2

Prevention in the Family And the Community

Most of us don't want young teens pushed into early sexual activity as a result of peer pressure, ultimatums given by a boy/girlfriend, or exploitation. We would like teens to abstain from sexual intercourse until they're truly ready to support a family—ready emotionally, physically, psychologically, and financially.

Most of us would agree the best way to avoid the problems of too-early parenting is for teenagers not to become pregnant until they're equipped for the responsibilities of parenthood. Preventing teenage pregnancy is an important part of the "solution" of a lot of problems before they happen. This is where the teen pregnancy prevention continuum begins.

No longer do we have a chaperone culture. Saying "No" to sex in our culture means making an individual and conscious decision to resist the messages so prevalent from music, media, bumper stickers, advertising, and peers to "do it." It means not following the many role models along this line from Hollywood to our home towns.

Saying "No" requires high self-esteem and a sense of self at a level even many adults haven't achieved. It requires having future goals and a realization that those goals are obtainable. Saying "No" requires that little girls learn to be independent and sure of their own futures, and that little boys understand that they can prevent pregnancy just as well as girls can. It requires that little boys learn a sense of responsibility and caring, and the understanding that becoming a man doesn't involve fathering a baby one can't support. Neither does it mean pressuring someone into sexual intercourse just to say he's "done it."

It would be wonderful if little boys and little girls gained these feelings of self respect, independence, responsibility, and caring within their homes from their parents. In many families, this happens. Within other families, families already mired in hopelessness, children may not develop these characteristics without a great deal of community help.

While the family is or should be the primary center for information and education about sexuality behavior, the community has historically played a crucial role in supporting family efforts. We know that families have never been able to do it by themselves. The community has always played a vital role in support of families and helping kids deal with the many problems of growing up.

It is imperative that we continue to provide this help. More and more we're realizing that teenage pregnancy prevention involves far more than teenagers refraining from sexual activity, or the use of contraceptives by those already sexually active. It involves teens having opportunities for success, developing feelings of self-worth, and having hopeful, healthy life options.

Efforts Directed Toward Prevention

More and more, local, state and national efforts are focusing on the prevention of too-early pregnancy. In designing a local prevention program, clarify what you mean by prevention. Are you talking only of primary prevention meaning abstinence? Or are you also talking about preventing teen pregnancy through contraceptive use by sexually-active youth? Don't get lost in semantics, but be clear about your program's goals.

Some activities and program initiatives simply target teen pregnancy prevention. Others link teen pregnancy prevention with the prevention of other adolescent at-risk behaviors, most notably substance abuse, school dropout, and suicide. Opinions differ regarding the linking of teen pregnancy prevention with other adolescent at-risk behaviors.

Pregnancy and parenting are positive concepts in our society, and it is only the timing that makes them undesirable for teens. The other at-risk behaviors, however, are not positive concepts at any time or for any age.

The development of self-esteem, career goals, decision-making skills, and the ability to say "No" to undesirable behavior, however, are an important part of too-early pregnancy prevention as well as prevention of other at-risk behaviors. These attributes are learned throughout an individual's development, from the cradle to adolescence, and throughout life.

Marie E. Mitchell, Director of the **Teen Services Program, Grady Memorial Hospital, Atlanta, Georgia**, shared a poignant anecdote. She was talking with a group of eighth graders about the reasons for delaying sexual intercourse and the need to be assertive in saying "No." A little girl in the class said, "I have two sisters. One had a baby when she was thirteen, and the other had one when she was fifteen. Until today I thought if a boy wanted to do it, that was what I was supposed to do."

Carol Cassell, author of *Straight from the Heart: How to Talk to Your Teenager About Love and Sex* (1987, Simon and Schuster) and co-author of *A Resource Book on Sexuality Education* (1989: Garland Press), writes:

> *While the causes of adolescent pregnancy are complex, we know that teen girls who have high self-esteem, a sense of being in control of their lives, and career ambition are unlikely candidates for pregnancy. Yet the association between female sex-role stereotyping, girls' lack of assertiveness, and teenage pregnancy is rarely made . . .*
>
> *It makes no sense that so many teen girls aren't being taught or expected to prepare for a world of accelerating*

economic and social change—unless you consider the
lingering residue of sexism in our culture (FLEducator,
Fall 1987, p. 3).

An extremely relevant issue in teen pregnancy prevention is
the sexism in our society. As long as little (and big) girls are
taught to be "nice," to be dependent, and as long as boys grow
up believing it's okay for them to sow their wild oats, too-early
pregnancy will continue to be one of the obvious outcomes.

Michael Carrera, noted sexuality educator, says, "'Just say
No' is just for girls. If we were targeting boys, we'd say, 'Don't
ask!'"

Many Different Goals for Prevention Programs

Teen pregnancy prevention programs, like care programs,
have many different focuses. Programs vary in their content and
target audience. Some are designed for a specific age. Some
target only males or only females. Some involve parents and
young people together. Others focus on the development of a
certain skill such as assertiveness techniques to resist peer
pressure or a characteristic such as self-esteem.

Probably the most exciting aspect of primary pregnancy
prevention programs is the number of exceptional local program
models which can be adapted for diverse settings. Also, in many
cases, the primary prevention activities may be less expensive to
start up and to maintain than some care programs would be.

Criteria for Prevention Programs

Since primary adolescent pregnancy prevention programs are
more diverse in content, in scope of services and activities, and
in the age of participants, the core criteria for successful programs may be difficult to define. Program professionals working
in primary prevention identified the following items as key
elements basic to a successful prevention program effort:

• **Comprehensiveness**
   Accurate, age-appropriate information.
   The availability of a full range of relevant educational,
      vocational, and life skills development opportunities.

The accessibility of support services such as adequate health care.

A diversity of activities that offer opportunities for personal success.

• **Program Atmosphere**

A comfortable, non-intimidating setting.

Facilitators who foster a feeling of open, honest communication and trust.

Strong emphasis on self-esteem, decision-making, and being responsible for one's actions.

• **Peer Group Support**

Offers a network for support.

Creates a sense of belonging.

Provides a forum for mutual problem-solving.

Provides encouragement and a climate for personal growth.

• **Parent and Community Support**

Effective prevention programs supported as a priority by parents and the community.

Parents and the community feel ownership in the program.

Consistent messages within the family and within the community reinforce the goals of primary prevention.

• **Individualization**

Provides for diverse levels of comprehension and maturity of participants.

Allows program provider to look at ways to enhance motivation, self-esteem, and self-sufficiency of each participant.

Provides opportunities for individual support and growth, often through a one-on-one relationship with an adult mentor.

• **Staffing—Employed or Volunteer**

Sensitive, caring, non-judgmental employed or volunteer staff.

Individuals who are comfortable with the program content and understand the stages of child and adolescent development.

Enjoy young people and have the ability to help them develop their skills and self-confidence.

- **Holistic Approach**

    Primary prevention services begin during the preschool
    years and continue through the teens by providing in-
    formation, skill-building opportunities, and a wide range
    of support services.

    Young people of all ages are treated as important parts of
    the program, of their families, and of their community.

    A wide range of opportunities are provided to enable
    participants to feel important and successful even
    in the smallest ways.

- **Funding Diversification**

    Need funding sources most likely to guarantee the stability,
    permanence, and expansion of the program.

    A long-range funding plan is developed from the start of
    the program.

    Staff is creative in looking for monetary or in-kind sources
    of local support.

- **Evaluation**

    Needs to be part of the initial program planning and
    implemented from the beginning.

    Utilizes a process appropriate and manageable for the
    specific program goals and one that measures the
    achievement of the program's desired outcomes.

    Successful evaluation findings are shared with program
    leaders, the funders, and the whole community.

Prevention Starts in Early Childhood

Good preschool programs may help prevent future untimely
pregnancies among participants. Long-range follow-up research
from the **Perry Preschool Program, Ypsilanti, Michigan,** for
example, shows the value of early childhood education for
preventing too-early pregnancy among children from
low-income families:

> *Preschool education led study subjects to lower fertility
> rates, as reported by age 19. Female study participants
> were asked how many times they had been pregnant and
> how many children they had at the time of the interview.*

Seventeen pregnancies or births were reported by the 25 women who had attended preschool; 28 pregnancies or births were reported by the 24 women who had not attended preschool. The difference between groups is statistically significant . . .; it corresponds to a pregnancy/ birthrate of 68 per 100 women for those who attended preschool, and 117 per 100 women for those who had not. (Changed Lives: The Effects of the Perry Preschool Program on Youths Through Age 19, page 69. 1984: The High/Scope Press.)

Emphasis on Parents of Preschoolers

Parents with coping ability, high self-esteem, and parenting skills are more likely to rear children with similar skills: children who have goals, children who will not have to make a baby in order to be somebody. A program indirectly promoting this goal for parents of preschoolers is **HIPPY,** the **Home Instruction Program for Preschool Youngsters.**

HIPPY was developed by the National Council of Jewish Women Research Institute for Innovation in Education at the Hebrew University of Jerusalem in Israel. It is a home-based program designed for under-educated parents to provide educational enrichment for their preschool children, thereby increasing parents' awareness of their own strengths and potential as home educators.

Support and training for the parents are given by para-professionals, themselves parents of young children, from the communities served by the program.

The first HIPPY programs in the United States were established in 1984. Today, approximately 2,400 economically disadvantaged families participate in programs operating in eight states. Miriam Westheimer, Director, HIPPY USA, explained:

Preventing teenage pregnancy is not one of our direct goals. HIPPY is planned for low socio-economic communities, rural and urban. A large percentage of the parents we serve are welfare recipients.

*It's important to teach children early. I also think it's
important to work with children through a model that
empowers parents. Many of the programs that take
children out of the home earlier and earlier tend to give
parents the message, "We can help your child, but you
can't." In the long run, this is not helpful.*

*Implementers of HIPPY are the parents. This says to
them, "You are your child's first educators. You know best
how to work with your child. We're giving you some tools,
but we aren't telling you that you can't teach."*

*We never assume that parents don't know and don't
care. We know they care about their children, but they
may not know how to get their kids ready for school.
Whether the school is at fault or the parents are at fault is
irrelevant. What we have is a program that will help
parents get their children ready to achieve at school.*

HIPPY parents allot time each day to working with their
children using packets of materials appropriate to their
children's developmental levels. Paraprofessionals visit each
parent at home every other week, bringing the storybook and
packet of activities for that week. Role playing is used to instruct
parents in the use of materials.

On alternate weeks, small groups of parents meet with their
paraprofessionals to review HIPPY materials, develop parent-as-
educator skills, and address other topics of special interest to
parents. These have included providing help with child-rearing
issues, learning to make toys and games, and getting information
about community programs in adult education or job training.

HIPPY materials are not lesson plans for professional educators, Westheimer stressed. They are designed to provide parents
who have had little (and often unsuccessful) formal education
with the necessary structure to implement a school readiness,
home instruction program. The activity packets concentrate on
language development, sensory and perceptual discrimination
skills, and problem solving.

Teenage mothers could be a significant part of the HIPPY
population. Parents become the HIPPY paraprofessionals, and

this often is their first work experience. "By the time a woman has worked with this program for two or three years, her skills increase tremendously," Westheimer said.

Preliminary research findings suggest that HIPPY has important positive impacts on participating mothers by improving their overall self-concepts and by increasing their interest and involvement in the education of their children, their involvement in community affairs, and their interest in pursuing further education for themselves.

HIPPY is an example of early intervention through the parents. It helps improve the self-esteem of both parent and child. The child who starts school with a zest for learning which began and will continue in his/her home is likely to continue learning, to set goals for him/herself, and to meet those goals. These are all important aspects of prevention of too-early pregnancy.

Helping Parents Talk About Sexuality

Key people in an agency or school are likely to support a sexuality education program for parents. A Board of Directors may need only to hear the rationale for parent programs and review a well-designed plan of action before approving such a program. Even if you've encountered opposition to sexuality education programs for teens in your area, you'll probably find that your community approves of parents being trained to communicate their own sexual values to their children.

We need to stress that a parent sexuality education program is not designed to change parents' attitudes or values. Instead, it is meant to help parents become more aware of their own values, and to develop the communication skills they need in order to convey those values to their children.

Probably the most essential factor in a successful course for parents is the teacher. S/he should have some knowledge of human sexuality, be able to discuss sexual topics with ease and comfort, and understand the tremendous responsibility of parenting. S/he will need to empathize with parents who are uncomfortable with discussion of sexuality. The teacher must also respect the diversity of values, and needs to support parents' right to teach their children the values in which they believe.

Ideally, the teacher will represent the major ethnic group of the parent participants. Educators working with parents of a different culture need to learn about and be sensitive to that culture. Presentations and materials used should reflect this sensitivity.

Session for Parents at Preschool

Because of the sensitive issues involved in human sexuality, many of us haven't developed the expertise we need in talking with our children about sex. Healthy sexual attitudes can be taught from birth, but often aren't.

Six Rivers Planned Parenthood, Eureka, California, includes sessions for parents of preschoolers in its community-wide **Family Life Education (FLE) Program**.

"We contact the preschools and set up a two-hour session for the parents," explained Mike Ware, Director of Education. "We show films, answer the questions and concerns the parents have about body parts, where babies come from, masturbation. We help them understand how talking to their kids at that age will help them be able to talk with them when they're teenagers."

Ware emphasized the importance of starting FLE programs with a strong coalition of parents and other community people.

See *Teen Pregnancy Challenge, Book One: Strategies for Change* (1989: Morning Glory Press) for a description of **Family TALKS,** another program for parents of preschoolers.

Bodies, Birth and Babies: Sexuality Education in Early Childhood Programs by Peggy Brick, et al (1989: **The Center for Family Life Education, Hackensack, New Jersey**) deals with the sexuality issues that arise in preschool. Brick authored the book with help from several directors of day care centers and a professor of early childhood education. Brick commented:

> *It became clear to us that this was needed when I was doing some training with preschool staff. There was nothing that addressed these issues. Everything written for little kids assumes the parents do it all, but now many*

children spend most of their waking hours in preschools.
Whether we think we're dealing with sexuality issues or
not, we give messages that either help or hinder them in
feeling okay about being a boy or being a girl, about
feeling good about their bodies.

Sol Gordon, widely known sex educator and author of
Raising Your Child Conservatively in a Sexually Permissive
World (1986: Simon and Schuster), believes the best approach
for little kids is educating them and promoting self-esteem.
Parents need to say, "Nothing will happen to you that will be
made worse by talking to me about it."

Research reveals that young people whose parents talk to
them about sex are the ones who delay their first sexual experience, and when they have sex, they use contraception, Gordon
pointed out. He continued:

The plain fact is that knowledge is not hormonal.
People who are knowledgeable are the people who think
before they act. Those without knowledge or those who
are into spontaneity—they are the ones who say "It's so
romantic just to let it happen." They're the ones who say,
"I didn't plan it so it's not my fault." We need to stress
that the people who aren't knowledgeable are the ones
getting pregnant.

Middle Childhood Prevention Efforts

The **"DARE To Be You" (Decision-making, Assertiveness,
Responsibility, Esteem)** program is a primary prevention
activity for pre-adolescents (eight-twelve years old) and their
parents.

The program focuses on the primary prevention areas of self-
esteem, decision-making, communication skills, and self
responsibility, as well as development of strong family support
systems. Sexuality is not directly addressed in the DARE
program.

Adults and teens interested in using the program may train to
become DARE group leaders, working directly with youth in
schools, other organizations, or within the home.

Developed by Janet Miller-Heyl, Health Specialist with the Colorado State University Cooperative Extension Service, the prevention program is adaptable to many groups in a local community setting.

Marilyn Lanphier, Director, Adolescent Health Section, Oklahoma State Department of Health, directs the DARE program in that state. She explained:

> *The DARE program works well in many community settings. It gives parents and children a positive way to communicate about the difficult issues related to growing up.*
>
> *We chose this curriculum because it dealt with a number of factors that impact on teen pregnancy. We wanted to change the "It just happened to me. I have no control over my life" kind of thinking. We wanted parent involvement because the schools certainly can't do it all, and health facilities can't do it all. It's also an inexpensive program which means we can implement it with more kids.*

Focus on Mothers/Daughters

The **Mother-Daughter Choices** program was developed through the **Girls Club of Santa Barbara** for sixth grade girls and their mothers. Mother-daughter pairs meet with a mother-coordinator for six two-hour meetings, often in the homes of participants.

Sessions consist of selected activities taken from *Choices: A Teen Woman's Journal for Self Awareness and Personal Planning* and the adult companion book, *Changes: A Woman's Journal for Self Awareness and Personal Planning*. Mothers are encouraged to start the program in their communities with the help of a handbook and a two-hour training video.

Purpose of the program is to prepare girls for the kinds of decisions they will be making as they move into young adulthood. Major goals are to encourage communication between mothers and daughters, and to help build girls' capacities for becoming economically independent.

Prevention for Teen Parents' Siblings

At the **Teenage Parent Program (TAPP), Louisville, Kentucky**, the staff has always been aware that teenage pregnancy is a situation that involves the entire family unit, according to Georgia Chaffee, principal. Utilizing the evening hours, the TAPP Family Programs offer counseling, support, and education to meet the needs of all family members. This program receives funding from foundations, grants, and private donations.

The Siblings Program, created as a pregnancy prevention strategy for brothers and sisters of TAPP students and Fatherhood Program participants, is an important component. The children are divided into age groups (six-eight years old, nine-eleven, twelve-sixteen) and are involved in activities that build positive self-image and confidence. The goal of the Siblings Program is prevention of both negative behavior and premature pregnancy.

"These children find themselves in a difficult situation as the family focuses on the new pregnancy. Siblings come to TAPP and express their feelings concerning their options," Chaffee explained. Sara York, TAPP Family Programs Coordinator, described outreach activities with the Siblings Program:

> *We're doing a lot of home visits. We're also doing school visits, speaking with the children's counselors, really concentrating on the positive.*
>
> *Sometimes a female sibling gets pregnant to regain her parents' attention. She's feeling resentment or jealousy because her pregnant sister is getting so much attention, whether positive or negative. What we're trying to do is to communicate to the youngsters that they do not have to act out or get pregnant in order to get attention.*
>
> *In one session with six- to eight-year-olds, the instructor led an activity based on Peter Pan. A little girl said, "I wish I was Peter Pan because I don't ever want to grow up and be like my sister, and have a baby."*
>
> *That, of course, opened the door for the instructor to say, "Well, there are good things about your sister, but*

let's talk about the things you can do so you don't become pregnant until you're ready."

Junior High/Parent Program in Churches

Frequently people who work with pregnant and parenting teens choose to add a prevention program to their services. Mary Shafer and Sharon Lockwood are co-directors of **The Bridge**, a support program for single mothers in **Fargo, North Dakota**.

With assistance from other professionals interested in working on prevention, Shafer and Lockwood developed a four-week session for junior high youth and their parents, the **Family Life Enhancement Series**.

Other professionals in the community do much of the teaching of body awareness and other physical issues, self-esteem, adolescent pregnancy and decision-making, and relationship issues.

"Our overall goal is to promote communication about sexuality between parents and teenagers because research shows that when parents and kids talk, pregnancy is less likely to happen," Shafer explained.

The Family Life Enhancement Series is generally done through the churches. "We're a very conservative state, and marketing anything dealing with sexuality is difficult here," Lockwood remarked.

"The pastors invite us to present this as part of their confirmation classes, and we invite the pastors to be there with us. What we do is acceptable to almost any church. If they want to add a section on contraception, we do it. If they don't want it, we don't include it.

Actually, we haven't gotten any negative reactions, probably because our program is church-sponsored."

"We do this as volunteers," added Shafer. "For a short time, there was state money available, but that ran out, and we decided to continue anyway. Everyone involved is mostly volunteering their time. The church usually donates money to print a brochure, and they duplicate our handout materials. We're real low budget. You don't have to have a lot of money to do something."

Lockwood and Shafer have been presenting the Family Life Enhancement Series for several years, usually four or five times each year, with attendance ranging from twenty to one hundred. "The churches usually ask us to come back," Lockwood concluded.

Comprehensive Program for Teens, Parents

The Children's Aid Society conducts programs at three locations in **Central Harlem.** These innovative pregnancy prevention programs involve the unlikely inner-city program components of tennis, golf, and squash.

Too many pregnancy prevention programs focus on the "narrow genital dimension" of sexuality and fail to address the fundamental reasons for teenage sexual activity and pregnancy, according to Michael Carrera, director of the innovative **Dunlevy-Milbank Teenage Pregnancy Prevention Program.**

The key to preventing teenage pregnancy, he maintains, is to persuade young teenagers to delay sexual intercourse by giving them confidence that they are important and are capable of achieving worthwhile goals. Dr. Carrera believes holistic programs must be developed and sustained over many years in order for change to occur in the lives of the youngsters and families.

There are seven dimensions to the program:
1) A fifteen-week on-going series on family life and sex education involving the teens and their parents.
2) Individualized, lifetime sports such as squash, swimming, tennis and golf to encourage self-discipline and impulse control.
3) Creative expression and performing arts to enhance self-esteem.
4) Career awareness, job preparation and employment through the Job Club.
5) On-going health and medical services designed to meet the needs of adolescents.
6) Academic support program—homework help, tutoring, and guaranteed admission to Hunter College.
7) Individual and family counseling.

Initially funded by the New York State Department of Social Services Teenage Pregnancy Program, the program also involves the Junior League for tutoring and homework help. During the first year, the program worked with a core group of fifty-five teenagers (thirty males, twenty-five females) and twenty-seven parents of these youths (mostly single mothers).

At the end of the first year, not one of the girls had become pregnant, and not one of the boys had caused a pregnancy. At the end of two years, with seventy-five participants (forty males, thirty-five females), there had been only one pregnancy in an area where approximately one girl in three is pregnant by age eighteen. During the first five years, there were only two pregnancies among the females and one male had caused a pregnancy, according to Carrera.

PACT Program Developed in Montana

The Parents and Adolescents Can Talk (PACT) program was developed through the Department of Home Economics, and now is provided through the Cooperative Extension Service at Montana State University in Bozeman.

PACT is a community-based communication and sexuality education program for adolescents/pre-adolescents and their parents. Partially funded through a grant from the Office of Adolescent Pregnancy Programs (OAPP/DHHS), the family-oriented program was created by a group of parents, clergy, health care, agency, and education personnel.

The training program has been designed in separate curricula—one for fifth and sixth graders, one for seventh through ninth graders, and one for tenth through twelfth graders, each to be used with the student's parents.

The material is divided into a series of lessons focusing on self-esteem, parent-adolescent communication, assertiveness, decision-making and knowledge, values, and attitudes toward sexuality.

Designed to be used in many types of community settings, a primary purpose of the program is to help parents reclaim their responsibility as the primary sex educators of their children, and to facilitate family communication on sexuality issues.

The program is not limited to Extension Service sponsorship, and no new organizational structure is needed, according to Joye Kohl, professor at MSU and director of the program's development. However, someone must provide key leadership. That someone can be a clergyperson, a 4-H leader, school administrator, hospital personnel, or someone from a social service organization.

Cost of the program is low because the facilitators are usually either community volunteers or persons already being paid by their agencies. The curriculum is available from the PACT Program in Montana, and it has been implemented in many states. Training is available from PACT but is not required for facilitators.

"We were always committed to the family approach. Parents don't get the credit they deserve in this area. It's not that they don't want to talk with their children, but rather the fact that parents often lack the skills, the vehicle, and the confidence for doing so," Kohl asserted. "Parents continually told the facilitators, 'It's nice to know that other parents have the same concerns.'"

Another parent commented, after participating in PACT, "We spend time teaching our children how to drive when they reach the proper age. Surely it's worth time and money to teach our children how to 'drive' their bodies properly to mature and healthy adulthood."

Providing Outreach to Schools

Inwood House in New York City is a human services agency serving young, single women and their children since 1830. Since 1971, its clients have been almost entirely pregnant teenagers and teen mothers. Inwood House provides maternity residence care, joint foster care for teen mothers and babies, and aftercare services for those returning to community living.

The Inwood House Community Outreach Program, also known as **Teen Choice**, is a model program of adolescent pregnancy prevention conducted in selected New York City junior and senior public high schools. Students attending these schools live in high risk areas.

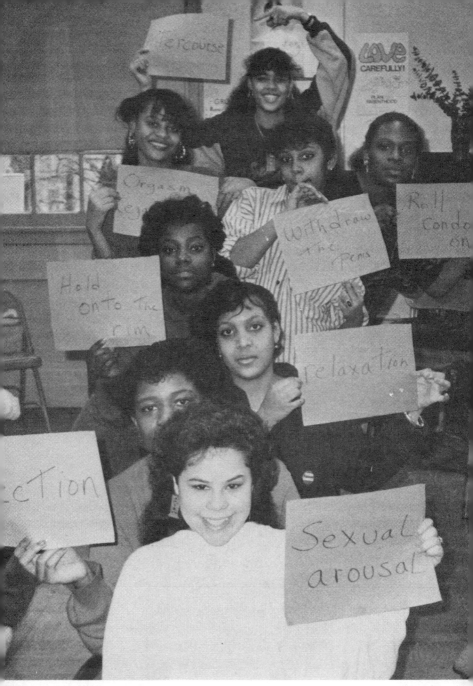

Teen Choice group
Inwood House Community Outreach

Information, counseling, and referral on human sexuality, fertility management, pregnancy, and parenting are offered to teenage boys and girls in school settings. Teen Choice helps adolescents make informed and responsible choices regarding their sexuality. The Teen Choice program takes a stand on issues without being judgmental of individuals who choose different values, according to Mindy Stern, Director, Community Outreach Program. She described the program's value base:

- Being a teen parent is not a good idea. It brings with it many social, emotional, educational, financial, and medical problems.
- No one should be pressured into a sexual act against his or her will or against his or her principles.
- The double standard for males and females, which still exists in our society, is not to be condoned.
- Postponement of sexual intercourse is encouraged until after high school or until marriage.
- If a couple decides to have sexual intercourse, they should always use birth control/safer sex practices.

Through individual counseling, group counseling, and classroom presentations, teenagers are helped to understand the reproductive cycle, to explore values, and to become more aware of the physical and emotional consequences of their behavior. This program encourages and supports those teenagers who choose to postpone sexual activity.

Teen Choice helps sexually active adolescents who either wish to use, or are using birth control to maintain consistent, effective usage. Pregnant girls and young parents are offered information and counseling about health, finances, and child care options so they may continue their education while caring for their own and their babies' physical and emotional needs.

An outreach social worker is placed in each participating school and works closely with school staff and cooperating agencies such as neighborhood health care clinics and the borough-based Teen Pregnancy Networks. Social workers develop referral linkages with medical and social services, provide training, and act as consultants to school faculty and other professionals in the field on issues relating to teenage sexuality.

Teen Choice is sponsored by the New York City Board of Education's Office of Alternative High Schools and Programs, High School Division. Funding is provided by grants from private foundations and the New York City Youth Bureau.

Wide Variety of Programs Needed

Prevention of too-early pregnancy takes many directions. Good preschools and parent programs such as the HIPPY at-home program are examples of early intervention. Community programs for elementary children and their parents, programs provided through the churches, health services, and youth organizations, play a big role in helping children move into adolescence with healthy attitudes toward their bodies and their role in society. Programs for adolescents and for their parents help young people develop the attitudes and the skills they need to delay sexual intercourse as they work toward productive futures.

Hundreds of other programs designed to help youth delay too-early sexual activity are in operation across the country. Hundreds more are needed.

CHAPTER 3

Primary Prevention— In the Schools

We give our schools a great deal of responsibility in educating our children, and many of us believe that responsibility also includes teaching that is designed to prevent premature pregnancy. Our children need a collaborative network of support from their families, their churches, their communities, and their schools on this issue as well as the many other issues affecting their lives.

Parents are the first and most important sexuality educators for their children. Ideally, children will gain from their families a sense of self-worth, respect for themselves and others, and the ability to set goals for themselves and to achieve those goals. They will learn a healthy and responsible attitude toward their own sexuality. However, parents aren't the sole educators of their children. Churches and community organizations may also be involved.

But that's still not enough. Bottom line—schools are where the kids ARE! It's where their peers are. When we're educating the peer group, we may have a better chance of having our message heard and understood.

Community Service Program for Students

One approach to involving teens within their communities through their schools is the **Teen Outreach Program**. This school-based program for adolescents is designed to decrease teen pregnancy and increase the number of teenagers who successfully complete their education by placing teens as weekly volunteers in community agencies.

In addition to their volunteer experience, teens of both sexes participate in weekly small group discussions led by a trained facilitator/teacher who guides them through a curriculum focusing on life management skills. The curriculum includes discussions and activities centered around such topics as self-esteem, values, communication, human growth and development, families, relationships, and parenting.

Initially promoted and funded by the Junior League of St. Louis, Teen Outreach is now directed by the **Association of Junior Leagues** national office. Funding from the Charles Stewart Mott Foundation enables the replication of the program in local communities across the country.

Marilyn Steele, Program Officer of the Mott Foundation, explained the program further:

> *We know that education alone is not an antidote to changing human behavior. It must be based on an intervention strategy. With that awareness, the Mott Foundation decided to fund the Teen Outreach Program for high-risk young men and women.*
>
> *The issue of healthy self-concept is basic to most social programs dealing with youth. Dealing with one's own sexuality and being able to identify as a sexual being is an important part of that goal. In addition, young people need access to and knowledge of contraceptives.*
>
> *Teen Outreach is an after-school model that offers this kind of curriculum using a teacher who moonlights after school, someone who is paid to work with high-risk boys*

and girls, usually ninth or tenth graders. Teen Outreach also provides a volunteer work experience for these young people. For many of them, this is the first time in their lives that they see themselves as caring for someone else— child care, working with the elderly, assisting in a hospital or recreation program.

These two characteristics—informal curriculum in a discussion group and appropriate work in a human services agency—seem to provide high payoff. With four years of evaluation, we know that, in terms of staying in school and reducing pregnancy and childbirth rates, young people in the program are doing substantially better than are comparable young people not there.

The program is growing. Currently it's being supported in thirty communities across the country.

"Teen Outreach is an easy program to replicate," commented Wendy McNeil, Coordinator, Adolescent Pregnancy Program, Association of Junior Leagues. "Find a school willing to partici- pate, find a teacher willing to teach the course, and find an organization willing to work with the school, and you're ready to start." The organization can be the Junior League or any other volunteer agency which can identify community service programs in which the kids can participate.

The Mott Foundation's grant goes to the Association of Junior Leagues to coordinate the overall programs, while local dollars support the local Teen Outreach. This is a low-cost program, according to Steele, because it's organized by volun- teers. "It costs less than $10,000 for twenty-five participants per year, and volunteer organizations like Kiwanis and Rotary can make contributions. A few contributors can support Teen Outreach for a school year if the school can contribute the teacher's salary after the school day," she explained.

Student Panels Teach Prevention

Many schools and other organizations use teen panel presen- tations as a pregnancy prevention technique in schools and other youth groups. Non-parenting youth may be recruited as peer educators as in the **Postponing Sexual Involvement** program in **Atlanta, Georgia.** In other programs, panels of teen parents share some of the hardships and real life experiences of early parenting.

In Tennessee, however, sexually abstinent youth and teen parents are combined in panels for the **Chattanooga Adolescent Awareness Team (CHAAT).** Pamela Wild, Coordinator, provides a thirty-hour training program for these young people, half of which includes sex education and the other half, public speaking training. Students are paid minimum wage during the training, and slightly more after completion.

"We talk to schools, youth groups, and churches, and we're offering our services to professional groups—nurses, social workers, civic organizations, PTAs," explained Wild. "The young people talk about their lives, usually focusing on aspects they and their audiences feel are especially important. The main purpose is to promote abstinence and sexual responsibility."

"We have males and females, both abstinent and teen parents. People respond favorably, especially abstinent girls who say it's nice to know they aren't alone," she concluded.

The CHAAT panels recently have been doing more and more presentations to adult groups. According to Wild, these are the result of evaluations indicating CHAAT teens are good role models for parents, too, on how to speak openly and honestly about sexuality.

Gaining Support for Family Life Education

For some communities, family life education (FLE) is a divisive issue. Parents may be concerned that the school is taking away the family's role as sexuality educators of their children. Involving parents in the planning and implementation of FLE programs is crucial.

Colusa County is a rural area in northern California. Three years ago the **Family Life Education Project** was funded with the goal of developing a family life education curriculum for the four school districts in the county.

Roberta Leggitt, Public Health nurse, was appointed Project Coordinator, and Harriett Jewett, Project Educator. Jewett is the parenting teacher in the local School Age Parent/Infant Development program.

Jewett and Leggitt's experiences in working on this issue with four very different and rather conservative communities provide insight into the difficult task of bringing together people with different viewpoints. Jewett shared their experiences:

We read 104 curricula, screened them, and the Advisory Board selected one for eighth grade. We took it out to each of the four communities, explained it to them, and asked them for input. I think that was the real strength of our project. We gave the Advisory Board a lot of power and our communities a lot of power.

At our Advisory Board meetings we reviewed all the comments for and against the program. We typed all the comments and sent them to the Advisory Board far enough in advance of the next meeting so they could read them and think about them. People on our Advisory Board were committed to children, but some were in favor of, and some were opposed to, having any family life education in the schools.

It was a long period of education. We educated the Advisory Board and the community about topics typically covered in family life education. They, in turn, educated us about their fears, which centered around teaching values clarification, the reproductive system, masturbation, birth control, abortion, and homosexuality.

One time, several Advisory Board members were leery of how we would be influencing young minds by teaching decision-making. So we demonstrated a lesson. When they saw what it was like in the real lesson, they didn't find it threatening.

Some of the people felt they did not want their eighth grade children making decisions. But as we talked, they began to understand that maybe they weren't allowing their children to learn how to make good decisions.

We (Advisory Board) finally agreed on the curriculum we liked. We had learned how different the communities were, so we provided options within the curriculum in the areas of consent process (parents' permission for child to participate in class) and the lesson on pregnancy alternatives.

One community turned down participating in the project and said they'd write their own. After several months of effort, they took our curriculum, changed the order of some of the material, and added some lessons. It's important in small communities for people to take ownership. At first we were leery of that, but it turned out well.

"Often, those who opposed us didn't have their children in the public schools."

In one town the school board had an Open Forum and allowed people to speak on both sides. The discussion was heated, but it seemed cleansing—everyone had their say. It helped the school board, it helped the town, and it helped us.

We had a twenty-four member board, very representative of the diversity in the community. It was exciting to see them because they came to meetings to work—they knew we'd listen to them.

We made copies of the curriculum available in the public library and at the schools so the public could read it.

Each time people who opposed our curriculum had meetings, we'd go. We wanted to know what was going on, but we didn't talk. We just listened. One minister, who opposed us in the beginning, asked to be on our board. He wound up promoting the curriculum.

At Advisory Board meetings the public was always invited to give input at the end. All we asked was that they give us their name, the school district where they lived, and where their children attended school. Often those who opposed us didn't have their children in the public schools.

*Parents have to know they're respected. This is impor-
tant. Sometimes they seem frustrated, but when someone
discusses the subject with them rationally, they understand. When people would argue in our public meetings,
we didn't try to combat the argument, but we did offer
information. Sometimes they'd go home and think about it,
and sometimes they changed their minds.*

*The best advice we got was from someone who said, "If
you listen to people, it makes a world of difference. Those
people who object always have valid reasons to object.
Their reasons may not be acceptable to you, but they are
valid reasons." When we started listening on that level, it
made all the difference.*

Sex Education in Parochial School

Jan Kern, President, Adolescent Pregnancy Child Watch, Los
Angeles, California, says the excellent Family Life Education
Program at her children's parochial school compliments her
involvement in the teen pregnancy issue. "My son came home
saying, 'Sister said sex is a gift from God,'" she reported.

Sister Stella Maria, Principal, **St. Paul the Apostle School,
Los Angeles,** believes firmly that boys and girls in her K-8
school of 530 students need guidance in learning about sexuality. "Catholic schools used to be very rigid and ever so proper,
but we're coming into the real world now," she remarked.

The school has been presenting sexuality programs for
several years. "The reason they've been successful is largely
because we've never done anything without consulting the
parents," Sr. Stella explained.

"We'd say, 'We're going to show this film on Thursday, and
we'd like you to see it on Tuesday night.' This took the threat
away for parents. It helped them understand that we know
they're the primary educators of their children."

Recently Sr. Stella offered an evening presentation to parents
and their fifth and sixth grade children, and another to parents
with seventh through eighth graders. "At both sessions we had
ninety-eight percent turnout of parents and children, and after-
ward I heard nothing but positive comments," she said. "I think

parents were nervous. Sometimes you could hear a pin drop, they listened so intently."

After seeing an appropriate film, children and parents at each session were invited to submit questions. Sr. Stella reported:

Questions were honest and upfront about dating, how a boy feels about a girl, and how a girl feels about a boy. But some of the parents were falling off their chairs because they had no idea their children knew as much as they did. Many of us can't talk about sex, and this program gave a common agenda for father and son, mother and daughter to start those discussions.

Most parents have common sense. You find a few who are a little nervous or a little conservative in their thinking. One or two parents said, "Oh, our kids are too young to know that. They don't need to know that every day three thousand teenagers get pregnant in the United States."

Other parents, however, say, "Yes, they need to hear that." In fact, one hundred percent of the parents signed permission for their children to participate in our sexuality classes.

A few of the parents wanted the religious issue covered, but we had to say, "No. These are simply facts, and we're imparting knowledge to children to help them make the right decisions."

PURPOSE Program for Parents

The Planned Parenthood Federation of America developed the **PURPOSE** program (Parents United for Responsible Policies on Sexuality Education). The program calls on parents actively to encourage the development of comprehensive school sexuality education programs in local communities because nationwide, only ten percent of all school-age children currently receive sexuality education in schools. Only thirty-five percent of American teenagers have received timely, comprehensive school sexuality education, according to Planned Parenthood.

PURPOSE is part of Planned Parenthood's comprehensive teen pregnancy prevention campaign. Affiliates nationwide are

organizing community PURPOSE steering committees to recruit parents to:
- Participate in intensive community-wide public education efforts to generate concern about sexuality education among friends and neighbors;
- Work with local school administrators and educators to develop and implement sexuality education curricula;
- Support federal, state, and local policy decisions that affect the sexuality education their children receive;
- Learn to give children the best possible tools to enable them to make responsible sexual decisions, and to make the most of their creative potential and reproductive future.

Family Life Education (FLE) Mandate

Almost ten years ago the New Jersey State Board of Education mandated family life education (FLE), including sexuality education, in the public schools. The state legislature expressed some opposition and modified some portions of the mandate, but New Jersey became the first state to require FLE. A process was developed by which the State Department of Education monitors local school districts for compliance.

Former Board member Susan N. Wilson, now Executive Coordinator of the **New Jersey Network for Family Life Education,** a research, advocacy, and technical assistance organization, reports that periodically a small band of opponents (about nine percent of the state's residents, according to a reliable poll) has tried to overturn or weaken the regulation. She commented:

I believe knowing about your body, your feelings and desires, and your sexual nature is critical to the normal process of growth and development. Even if there were no such social problem as teenage pregnancy, I think everyone needs to know and understand the ramifications of being a sexual being from birth to death. In order to accept our sexuality and behave in a responsible manner, all of us need information about that aspect of our lives.

Our free society is based for the most part on information. We crave correct, timely and thorough information

for all the other aspects of our lives, but, ironically,
sometimes refuse to honor the need for accurate and
complete information about the sexual aspects.

The New Jersey regulation as written involves parents as
partners in the provision of family life education. Each school
district must have a community advisory committee which
includes parent representatives. Parents receive an outline of the
FLE content for the grade in which their children are enrolled,
and can go to the district office to see materials. While they have
a right to remove their children from sessions which they feel
conflict with their religious or moral values, less than one
percent have done so.

Some schools in New Jersey offer FLE programs for parents.
"Many parents have not had the benefit of comprehensive
family life education during their own schooling and look to the
schools to assist their children," Wilson says. She points to
statewide polls that show overwhelming support (as high as
eighty-nine percent) for family life education programs in the
schools.

From her ten-year experience, Wilson believes that, while
the schools have a large role to play in providing instruction
about human sexuality, everybody should talk to young people
about the pleasures of being loving and sexual, and the
responsibilities, risks, and consequences that accompany it:

Parents, schools, churches and synagogues, and
community agencies should all be involved. Certainly
young people need plenty of information to overcome
media messages about sexual behavior that promises bliss
with no attendant risk or responsibility.

Perhaps children and adolescents will receive differ-
ent, contradictory messages from these different adults,
but they should be encouraged to think about what they
are hearing, helped to fit the messages into their develop-
ing system of values, and given skills to make decisions
about how to handle this aspect of their lives. Sexuality is
not something that happens only in puberty; it is an aspect

*of our lives that is always with us, and that grows and
changes.*

*Talking about sexuality is not harmful; talking does not
result in unplanned pregnancies or AIDS or date rape.
Talking, I believe, helps young people make better decisions. Is it fair for a teacher to refuse to answer a child's
question about sex with the comment that s/he should
consult her/his parents? Would the child ask the teacher
the question if the parents were able to provide the
answers?*

A comprehensive FLE program has three basic components,
according to Wilson::
- **Cognitive component** to provide facts;
- **Affective component** to give young people an opportunity
  to talk about attitudes and values;
- **Skills component** to help young people to think, to make
  decisions, to be assertive, to say "No," and to act responsibly and respectfully toward themselves and others.

Preparing Teachers for Mandated FLE

Kansas is another of the sixteen states now mandating that
school districts teach human sexuality and AIDS prevention to
elementary and secondary students. Betsy Bergen, Associate
Professor in Human Development and Family Studies at **Kansas
State University, Manhattan,** has taught human sexuality
courses for more than twenty years. Recently she has been
traveling throughout Kansas to help school districts meet the
Board of Education's mandate. She helps districts develop and
implement family life education programs, and she provides in-
service training for teachers.

"Some of our smaller communities are very, very conservative," Bergen commented. "In one community they said we
couldn't name the body parts until fourth grade—we couldn't
teach the words penis or vagina until then. Some cities don't
want us to talk about contraception other than abstinence, while
others say we need to give students the advantages and
disadvantages of each so they can make good choices.

"I have no objection to 'Just say No,' but I think that's a very limited approach to the problem, and apparently it hasn't worked in the past. I've been an educator for many years, and I think education presents a view and helps people make wise decisions. I don't know how we can help teenagers make wise decisions if we just say 'No,'" Bergen concluded.

Pamela Wilson, sexuality education consultant, Temple Hills, Maryland, stresses that sexuality education programs need to be comprehensive and age appropriate. She points out the impossibility of offering a comprehensive program in a one-week course.

Wilson recommends training classroom teachers to be comfortable and knowledgeable about the subject, then fitting FLE curriculum units into various classes, such as social studies, health, and science, throughout the year.

"Teachers already are dealing with family topics such as communication," she pointed out. "Sometimes the sexuality curriculum can be built on the foundation of subjects already taught in some classrooms. This makes more sense than doing it out of context for three weeks."

The danger in this approach, according to Wilson, is that some teachers may not infuse the FLE units into their existing curriculum. "The highly motivated and excited teacher will do it, but the others may only present units with which they feel completely comfortable. For these teachers, being told to teach FLE at a specific time might work better."

"There has to be a strong mandate from the school administrator, the principal, or the superintendent. Teachers have to understand it is not optional. If this isn't done, some teachers won't teach it," she added.

Wilson feels the climate for effective family life education is becoming more positive:

> *Sexuality education is important because it helps people understand themselves. Our most important goal in FLE is to be prepared for the developmental changes we all experience. Another goal is to understand ourselves and our feelings, to know that a range of feelings in all*

kinds of situations are natural and normal, but that feelings don't have to be acted upon.

Another important goal of sexuality education is to understand that sexuality is natural and an important part of being human. It's still looked at as this tiny aspect of life, and kids are not comfortable talking about it. They're talking about it all the time, but not in healthy, positive ways.

Kids are pressured in ways we were never pressured, and I think we have to give them the comfort and the skills to talk about sexuality in meaningful ways, and to assert themselves. I think with comprehensive programs throughout the country, we could have a generation of parents who could talk comfortably with their children about this issue. I think this would be fabulous.

School-Based Health Clinics Since 1967

The red flag goes up in some communities when the possibility of opening a school-based health clinic is mentioned. Yet in Dallas more than twenty years ago (1967), two school-based clinics were opened on elementary school campuses. These clinics were organized through the Dallas Children and Youth Project, Department of Pediatrics, University of Texas Health Science Center at Dallas. They served a low-income area in West Dallas.

Based upon positive health outcomes at the two pediatric clinics, the **Children and Youth Project** was approached to help address the problem of excessive high school absences due to medical and psychosocial concerns.

Because the large adolescent population of the area was not being served, a clinic was established at Pinkston High School in West Dallas. Later evaluation showed a significantly lower adolescent pregnancy rate at this school compared to a similar school in the same city.

The well-staffed **West Dallas Youth Clinic** continues to offer health care to young people in the area.

Truman Thomas, now Executive Director of Impact, Inc., Dallas, was director of the West Dallas Youth Clinic during its early years. He commented:

Our total focus back in 1968 was on health care for children and adolescents in order to reduce the morbidity and mortality. We were in an area where parents couldn't afford to miss a day of work to take their children to a clinic. We could serve them during school hours on the school campus, so we said to the parents, "We need your permission because by law we can't treat your child without it." That was the way it started.

"A school-based clinic is not likely to get static in neighborhoods with a medical shortage."

We called parents and explained the concept of total health care. Parents would say, "This is a good deal. Sure, I'll sign the permission form."

When we started, we didn't dispense contraceptives. Then the community said, "You really need to do something about adolescents getting pregnant. You need to be more comprehensive," so we started providing birth control in 1971.

There was no static at all when we opened. A school-based clinic is not likely to get static in neighborhoods with a medical shortage. In those communities many of the problems would be solved if young people could get adequate health care, and it's in those communities where parents are willing to stand behind the clinics. When a clinic does meet resistance, for the most part I believe it's caused by outsiders trying to impose their values.

Last year about fifteen percent of the total population used the clinic for family planning services. We know that from the time the clinic opened in 1970 until 1980, the teen pregnancy rate in that particular area decreased thirty-three percent.

We can't say it was entirely because of the clinic because there were a lot of state and federal programs in place during that time, but the clinic was the consistent entity. We had a population across town that we used as

*a comparison group, and in that group, the pregnancy
rate went up.*

*Since 1980 we haven't had the resources to keep
gathering data. Also, since about 1978, we've lost so
many programs here, and our services have had to be cut
so much that we know we're less effective.*

*We like to think, "If we offer family planning services,
that will reduce the pregnancy rate," but it's really the
whole menu, the whole conglomerate of all the different
services, psychological issues, social issues, relationship-
building issues, primary health care, making one feel
better about oneself, all in addition to family planning
issues. To make a difference, we need to provide services
in all these areas.*

Community-Wide Effort Has Big Impact

Five years of public health information and education intervention in the Denmark-Olar School District #2, South Carolina,
has resulted in a statistically significant lowering of the rate of
adolescent pregnancy in the area.

Messages emphasizing the development of decision-making
and communication skills, self-esteem enhancement, and
understanding of human reproductive anatomy, physiology, and
contraception were targeted at parents, teachers, ministers and
representatives of the churches, community leaders, and children
enrolled in the public school system. The rate of pregnancy in
the area for females aged fourteen to seventeen years has
declined remarkably since the intervention began. These
changes are statistically significant when compared with three
similar counties, and also with the eastern portion of the target
county.

**The School/Community Program for Sexual Risk
Reduction Among Teens** was started in October, 1982, with
funding from the Office of Adolescent Pregnancy Programs
(OAPP/DHHS). At the end of the five-year grant, the state
picked up the funding. The county has a homogeneous rural, low
income, and under-educated population. In 1980, fifty-eight
percent of the county residents were black and forty-two percent

were white. There is little migration into or out of the county. The economy is primarily agricultural, and there is no public transportation.

Before the Sexual Risk Reduction program began, the county was among the top twenty percent of forty-six South Carolina counties in estimated pregnancy rate (EPR). EPR equals live births plus fetal deaths plus induced abortions for women aged fourteen through seventeen. The EPR declined from sixty per thousand before 1982 to twenty-five per thousand in 1984 and 1985. In the three comparison counties with no intervention program, EPRs increased during this period.

Instrumental in these results was the education of adults in the target community. School district teachers are offered three tuition-free university graduate-level courses related to sex education. Two-thirds of the district teachers, administrative staff, and special services professionals have completed at least one of these three-credit courses.

These trained teachers, assisted by project staff, implemented sex education in kindergarten through grade twelve and in all subject areas, using an integrated curriculum approach. They have no specific sex education course. Instead, teachers integrate units of instruction within their biology, science, social studies, and other courses.

Clergy, church leaders, and parents are also continually recruited to attend mini-courses addressing the same objectives as those developed for the schools. The primary goal for these adults is to improve their skills as parents and as role models for youth in the community.

In addition, program staff promote program objectives through the local newspaper, radio station, and speakers bureau. These community awareness activities have a broad-based health focus, and are not always specifically sex-related. Alcohol and drug abuse, nutrition, weight control, and smoking are highlighted.

Generic to all activities is the emphasis on problem solving— considering alternatives, assessing risks and consequences, making informed choices, and assuming personal responsibility for the outcomes of one's actions.

The results of this community education program offer conclusive evidence that intervention can indeed cause a decrease in the rate of teenage pregnancy within a community. Charles Johnson, Project Coordinator of the School/Community Sexual Risk Reduction Program for Teens, shared some techniques for involving a community in such a program:

> *Whatever you do must involve collaboration of school and community people. It's easy to talk about the schools doing it by themselves or the churches being responsible, but everybody has to be on the same wave length if you really want to reduce teenage pregnancy.*
>
> *How do you get the community involved? You go to a lot of churches. You go to a lot of meetings. You become a friend, you do everything in your power to be a part of the community. You have to be caring and concerned. You don't start out talking about contraceptives. You go into a church, for example, and you start talking about teenagers' problems. Talk about adolescent health—in every age group, life expectancy has increased except that of people aged fifteen to twenty-four. When you do this, you are setting the stage for parents to understand we aren't talking about an isolated problem. We're talking about a series of problems.*
>
> *Gradually you move on to a discussion about teenage pregnancy and how it's been a problem with us for years. You share some facts about the rates of pregnancy in the country, the state, and especially the local community. With a step-by-step approach, they understand the issue much better. They understand that when young girls drop out of school, it's a financial as well as a social burden.*
>
> *We're a rural area, and sex is a highly charged controversial subject. One must proceed carefully. First of all, we're trying to help kids develop skills to avoid becoming sexually active. The community accepts this goal.*
>
> *Second, once the teenager is sexually active, what do you do? This is a difficult subject for many people, so focus has been on primary prevention and getting parents*

and teens to work together. We know many teens are
sexually active, but when we focus on that, it polarizes the
issue, and parents think the program is corrupting their
children. You can't win that argument. Lots of good
parents think that giving children information on
contraceptives is encouraging promiscuity.

Of course we talk about contraceptives, but you can't
repeat that so much that people think that's all you're
*about. This is a critical point, and **how** you explain what*
you're doing is important.

Involve Entire Community

Kathy, a senior when her baby was born, would have appreciated the services offered in the above district. She feels her
school is failing teenagers in the area of sex education:

They don't have any sex education here except health.
There needs to be more talk about teen pregnancy and
how hard it is to have a baby. I think we should talk about
birth control, and I think they should give out contracep-
tives. It would be more fair to kids because it's tough,
really tough having a baby.

Schools alone cannot solve the problem of too-early pregnancy, but they can be an important part of the solution by
working in partnership with parents, agencies, and other segments of the community. In most areas, schools are where the
majority of kids spend nine months of every year for thirteen
years. That time frame allows programs to work with young
people in a significant way over an extended period of time.
That's important because intervention over a period of time is
far more likely to be effective than is a brief series of meetings
with young people.

It is important that we not leave adolescent pregnancy prevention only to the schools, or to the community, to the
churches, or even to the family. Teen pregnancy prevention is a
challenge to be confronted in each of these settings. It is a
challenge that requires intervention from all of us. Only then can
we hope truly to make a difference in young people's lives.

CHAPTER 4

Working with Sexually Active Teens

Most of us would prefer that young women and young men in their early teens not become sexually active. Cognitively, developmentally, and emotionally, many adolescents are not ready for the responsibilities of sexual intercourse.

We know, however, that about half of the teens in the United States are sexually active by age seventeen. Of course we support abstinence, but if we only stress "Just say 'No,'" we're missing a large group of young people. Programs targeting sexually active youth are needed.

Marie E. Mitchell, **Teen Services Program, Grady Memorial Hospital, Atlanta, Georgia**, feels that role modeling of adults push some teens into too-early sex:

> *Our teenage sexual behavior is mirroring adult sexual behavior right now. We think that how we manage our own sexual lives is right, and we cherish our freedom. If we choose to have sex without being married, that's all*

*right, and perhaps it is. But we need to remember that
young people model their behavior on ours. We're saying
this is the way our society is. We need to talk about that in
the classroom.*

*Many young people see their parents in dating rela-
tionships in which they know sex is involved. We tell kids
that yes, this may be true. But we also need to talk about
the different kinds of risks the young people may take, that
they have a choice to behave one way while other people
may make different decisions.*

Ellen Peach, co-author of **Family TALKS**, discussed the
relational reasons some young people are sexually active:

*We talk about kids getting sexually involved too early,
and we blame it on experimentation. But I think kids get
sexually involved for a lot of the same reasons adults do—
to be close, for some kind of affirmation, to be held, to feel
warmth from another human being.*

*So many of these kids are incredibly lonely. When we
work with sexually active teens, we can be more helpful if
we tune in to these needs. Adults tend to respond to the
early sex issue either by saying, "I don't want them to get
pregnant so let's give them contraceptives" or "Just say
'No.'" Because sexual activity among teenagers has
meaning above and beyond the act, getting in touch with
that meaning helps us have an idea as to how to deal with
that young person.*

*If they have been sexually abused, sexual intercourse
may be the only way they have learned to relate.*

*I think most of the young men have the same needs the
young women do, a need to feel connected, a sense of
belonging. Our society doesn't support that very well.*

Listen to the Teens

Peggy Brick, Director of Education, **The Center for Family
Life Education, Planned Parenthood of Bergen County,
Hackensack, New Jersey,** is the co-author of *Positive Images:*

A New Approach to Contraceptive Education (1987: Center for Family Life Education). When asked how she responds to the idea of telling teens, "Just say 'No,'" she said:

> *I tell them to talk to some teenagers. I feel if folks were in touch with teenagers, they would know how absurd "Just say 'No'" is. We talk to a lot of teens, and this absolutely turns them off.*
>
> *Furthermore, the "Just" is absurd. It takes a lot of self-esteem, a lot of self-control, a lot of standing up to peers to say "No." If we want them to say "No," we have to do a lot of sexuality education right from the start—preschool and kindergarten.*

Brick, who taught high school sex education for fifteen years, thinks more young people would choose not to have sexual intercourse so early if they could be involved in serious, open, non-judgmental, and non-moralizing discussions with adults. Brick continued:

> *I think we have to empower kids. We need to listen to teens tell us how we can help combat too-early pregnancy. I would like to put the kids into small rap groups with adults where they can talk about the pressures around them.*
>
> *Ask the adults about the messages in the media. What should we do, talk about it with the kids or let the messages go? What many adults are saying is out of touch with what kids are hearing all around them.*
>
> *Parents have to talk with their children and, even more important, listen to them. It's a process of listening to where the child is, what's bothering the child, and giving that child support. Children are exploited terribly through the media and advertising, and many parents aren't giving their children the support they need for saying "No." But the "Just say 'No'" thing is too glib, it's not relevant, and it's not coming from serious adults willing to address the issue with children.*

Another book by Brick, et al, *Teaching Safer Sex* (1989: The Center for Family Life Education), contains the following dedication:

> *To the young people of this nation*
> *Who must find their way*
> *To sexual health*
> *In a world of contradictions—*
> > *Where media scream, "Always say yes,"*
> > *Where many adults admonish, "Just say no,"*
> *But the majority*
> *Just say . . .*
> > *Nothing.*

Community of Caring Approach

The **Community of Caring,** a values-based curriculum developed by the **Joseph P. Kennedy, Jr., Foundation** for use in comprehensive programs serving pregnant and parenting teens, contains, among others, two teaching modules called "Putting Sex in Perspective" and "Family Development."

Lois H. Gatchell, long-time consultant on training with the Foundation and founder of the **Margaret Hudson Program, Tulsa, Oklahoma,** commented:

> *These modules help establish a base of factual informa-*
> *tion and a common vocabulary for talking about repro-*
> *duction and family planning. From these issues, the*
> *modules move on to emotional and cultural considerations*
> *so essential in a pluralistic society.*
>
> *Such areas as the differences between sex and love,*
> *relationships that exploit, the ingredients of a stable*
> *family, can then be explored.*
>
> *And in the process, if trust has been established, the*
> *teacher/counselor can reveal her values, and can encour-*
> *age the student to examine her personal values regarding*
> *love, marriage, and family.*
>
> *Many programs have found this approach helpful in*
> *their prevention counseling.*

Hotlines Provide Help

Ingrid Ligeon, Program Director of the **Eastern Virginia Pregnancy Hotline, Norfolk, Virginia,** feels that hotlines offer an important service in a community by providing a confidential and accurate information source.

The pregnancy hotline program started in 1984 through a cooperative effort between the state Department of Health and the Information Council of Hampton Roads (ICHR). At the time, ICHR provided a general hotline service for the southeastern part of the state. The pregnancy hotline was initially established as a place for pregnant women to call to get into prenatal care.

As soon as the hotline began operation in 1984, teens started calling with all types of questions related to pregnancy, contraception, and sexuality issues. The staff immediately redesigned the focus of the program to provide appropriate support and information for the adolescent callers.

Promotion for the hotline included the printing of TeenHelp cards, brochures, advertising in the school papers, and speaking to youth groups. As with many services for teens, the hotline staff found the best recruitment came from word of mouth.

Ligeon has some suggestions to share with groups interested in starting a hotline program:

> *First of all, the requested information needs to be given immediately. Don't put the caller on hold or have them call back or ask them to call another number. Information **must** be confidential.*
>
> *If possible, a pregnancy hotline for teens should link with an existing information service or with a program already serving adolescents. That facilitates outreach to possible clients.*
>
> *It's important that the teen callers feel confident and comfortable talking with the hotline staff. To be effective, you need to know the words the kids are using . . . and don't giggle. These issues are serious to teens, but they speak a different language than adults. I always get a language update from youth groups when I talk with them.*

Lastly, it's important to give the teen callers the same respect you would give an adult. Respect, a place to get confidential, accurate information, and someone to listen to their concerns—all are major reasons teens need a hotline service.

Accessibility Survey by Teens

In addition to the media's sexually-oriented messages and the lack of serious communication with adults, teens face other barriers to responsible decision-making.

Teen Council members of the **Center for Population Options (CPO)** recently conducted a contraceptive accessibility survey in sixty Washington, DC, drugstores. They uncovered a number of barriers teens face when purchasing contraceptives.

None of the drugstores surveyed displayed pamphlets discussing family planning methods. The survey revealed that stores often keep condoms behind pharmacy counters, making it necessary for teenagers to ask store personnel to retrieve them. When stores do display contraceptives in open aisles, more often than not, no sign marks the location.

Teen Council members then worked with the CPO staff in developing the text and format for a leaflet designed to help sexually active teenagers overcome the confusion and embarrassment they may experience when trying to buy and use condoms.

In cartoon format, "Advice from Teens on Buying . . . Condoms" covers how to find contraceptives in a typical drug store, how to choose the type of condoms that protect best against sexually transmitted diseases (STDs), and how to use a condom.

Clinic for Young Men

The Young Men's Clinic, Presbyterian Hospital in the City of New York, offers primary health care including sports and employment physicals, general illness treatment, and reproductive health care, including condom distribution.

About seventy percent of the young males (twelve to twenty-two years old) who come in are already sexually active, according to Bruce Armstrong, Assistant Clinical Professor, Center for Population and Family Health, Columbia University School of Public Health. Armstrong helped found the program.

Presbyterian Hospital is located in Washington Heights, a poor neighborhood with mostly Hispanic and African American residents including many recent immigrants. The area is sometimes identified as the crack capitol of the city, and it is medically underserved. During the Monday night clinic time, patients watch health education videos and participate in individual and group counseling. Much of the counseling is done by medical students who volunteer throughout the year so the clinic can personalize its health education delivery.

Armstrong described the clinic's beginning:

> *The kids told us if we labeled it a Family Planning Clinic or a VD Clinic, we wouldn't get them. If we made it more anonymous, we could meet their needs. Very few come in acknowledging they have questions related to their sexual activity. They may say they're having complexion problems or a stomach ache, but once they get here, it's easy for them to tell us about other issues that concern them.*

The Young Men's Clinic is relatively inexpensive to operate, Armstrong pointed out. Staff, in addition to him and several volunteers, consists of a full-time male coordinator of the medical/health education program plus a pediatrician one night each week.

An important factor in programs for men is having a catalyst to keep the profile high, according to Armstrong. In addition to working with young men, the coordinator visits the hospital's other reproductive health clinics which are held Tuesday and Wednesday nights. He conducts groups there which are composed mostly of young women. "Our concept is that there are many 'gatekeepers,' and you can get young men involved through their partners or their sisters. Since the women are coming in, we reach men through them," Armstrong observed.

When the Men's Clinic was started in 1985, a great deal of effort was spent on community outreach, Armstrong recalled:

We literally mapped it out—including parks, schools, after-school programs. We asked ourselves, "Who matters to the kids? Which coach can they trust?"

We knocked on doors everywhere, and sent out a lot of mail trying to sensitize people to the importance of involving young men. Some of the people we contacted, mostly adult men, bought into what we were doing and became our allies.

We became involved in several grassroots activities such as helping the kids clean up a park for a basketball tournament. Along with some of our medical students, we then helped them run their tournament for three summers.

We videotaped the boys playing basketball. We told them upfront who we were, then invited them to the hospital to watch themselves on tape and get sports physicals.

We don't do this as much any more because it is labor intensive, but it was very worthwhile in the beginning when nobody knew who we were. Now many kids come in to the Monday night clinic on their own because the word is out through the grapevine.

When you start a program, you have to find out where the kids are, and you have to go there to get them—and on their terms. If they need to meet at night, then meet at night. We did a lot of after-school work with the kids. They needed to see we were in tune with their culture. Basically, we tried to hook on to some of the good people and activities already in the community.

The Young Men's Clinic coordinator continues to keep in touch with community services by collaborating with other groups that work with young people, including groups which are mostly for young women. Armstrong explained:

You join and network with people who regularly provide a variety of services to young people. It's unfortunate that boys are so easily overlooked since efforts to involve them are much less expensive than services for the girls—condoms are not terribly expensive, and you don't need a physician to prescribe them.

For a relatively small amount of money, you can start so many ripples in motion. Every community organization can discuss issues of male involvement. If you take even a small part of your budget to hire a male to work with the men, you'll find it's cost-effective.

Male involvement is much more than condom use, however. We encourage our young men to bring their girlfriends in for foam, or they'll take a letter home saying "Withdrawal doesn't work," or "He's worried about you getting pregnant."

There is resistance to the idea of providing services for men. Family planning is still pretty much a woman-dominated field. Many people continue to have the idea that boys are not going to get involved, no matter how hard you try. But if you check into it, they aren't that way. We could tell story after story of the pressures they face to be sexually active.

Often boys feel embarrassed about using condoms because many young people really don't feel comfortable with what they're doing. I have had some male clients who have been more active in preventing pregnancy than have their girlfriends. We ought to show adults videotapes of boys' discussion groups so they could learn what the real concerns of young males are.

Involving young men is particularly important because AIDS has become such a big problem here. People are putting up less of a fuss about sexuality education because they realize it's better to be embarrassed than to die.

It's really not right to keep things under the table when we know young people may have several different partners. To put up so many barriers to these young people obtaining information and condoms is really questionable, especially in today's environment. I think you have to address these issues about sexual behavior directly without worrying that such discussion will stimulate them to go out and experiment. That's just not the case.

Working with High-Risk Youth

After coordinating Winston-Salem, North Carolina's Teen Talk for young women for two years, Beth Harris Brandes moved to Catawba County, North Carolina. Still with the Department of Social Services, she inherited **Teen Up,** a teen pregnancy prevention program for males and females. Because transportation appeared to be an unmanageable problem in this rural community, Brandes suggested going to the schools where they would have a captive audience.

She talked about the special challenge of working with high-risk youth:

> *We have targeted certain kids, those who have re-peated a grade, are known to be sexually active, exhibit other risk-taking behaviors such as substance abuse, truancy or court involvement, have been sexually abused, or demonstrate a sense of failure and/or depression. But I don't want them to be stigmatized.*

"They have a learned passivity
by the time they're ten or twelve
that terrifies me."

> *I don't say, "Your teacher said you should be here because you're sexually active." Instead, I ask them to be mature enough to handle the serious materials we'll be discussing, and second, I say the program is for kids who have had life experiences that have made them grow up fast.*
>
> *Then I say, "If you don't think you should be in this group, then please, you shouldn't be, and that's fine."*
>
> *I have never had a kid leave yet. It's important that we frame it in a way that gives them a choice. They're used to being singled out for negative reasons. I ask them to try the group for six weeks. Then if they want to continue, they must keep up with the class work they miss by coming to Teen Up. If they miss school more than one day a week, they must leave Teen Up. This pleases the principal.*

*I work with eighth graders now, and I see many kids
who feel they have no control over their lives. Building up
that idea of having choices is so important. They have a
learned passivity by the time they're ten or twelve that
terrifies me.*

*Last week in a group I led in the housing project, a girl
announced to the group that she wanted to get pregnant.
Someone said, "Why do you want to do that? You won't
get to go anywhere."*

"I don't get to go anywhere anyway," she replied.

*That hopelessness is tough to tackle. It's not going to
be solved in one session.*

Health Services for Rural Students

**The Adolescent Parent Prevention Program (APPP),
Snow Hill, North Carolina,** is a school-based clinic which was
started in 1982 in a rural area. Over the years, according to the
evaluation report (1982-1987), as a higher proportion of pregnant teens became APPP clients, the pregnancy rate, abortion
rate, and birth rate for teens decreased dramatically.

Helen Hill, Program Director since 1985, discussed setting up
the clinic and a follow-up teen survey. She recalls Elaine
Morgan, initial director, going, as a community health center
staff person, to the superintendent of schools and saying, "We'd
like to set up a school-based clinic out here which would
provide accessible health care for the kids."

"The kids were having real problems getting any kind of
health care," Hill related. "She told him our goal was also to
reduce teen pregnancy.

"He said, 'You aren't going to pass out contraceptives?'

"She said, 'No, sir, we're not.'" Contraceptives have never
been provided or prescribed at this clinic.

Hill continued:

*We started networking. We talked to the Department of
Social Services, Health Department, and other public
agencies. We told them the kids had to be educated, and
we wanted to do family life education in the schools. The*

superintendent had no problem providing the principals
gave their okay. So we met with all the principals, and
they agreed to our plan.

The parents were behind us too. Because a sixth grader
got pregnant about that time, parents were saying, "What
are we going to do about this?" That opened the door for
us because parents went to the school and said they had to
do something.

The clinic provides a wide range of health services. It is
located at the high school, but treats children at other
schools, too.

Three types of educational interventions were developed and
implemented, programs directed at three levels of prevention—
students who were not sexually active, students who were
considering the activity, and students who were already sexually
active. "Our number one way of dealing with prevention is
abstinence," Hill stressed.

A Family Life program was developed for grades five and
six. The Postponing Sexual Involvement (PSI) program was
implemented in both seventh and eighth grades. However, with
the onset of earlier sexual activity as shown by the teen survey,
PSI has been directed primarily to the seventh grade and
included in the sixth grade classes.

The last intervention, Teen Responsibility, was implemented
in grades ten through twelve, and later introduced in grades
eight and nine.

In 1985, a teen survey was conducted in grades seven
through twelve in the school district in order to gather baseline
data. The survey included knowledge, attitudes, and behavior
related to sex. The information provided the insight to target
more precisely program activities to meet the needs of the
adolescents. Hill explained how this happened:

In 1985 I went to the principal and the superintendent
and said, "I'm going to need some help from you all.
We're in our third year of funding, and I need to know if
what we're doing is making any difference. The only way I

can know that is to survey where the kids are in terms of
drugs, sex, various issues."

The report cards were going out a week later, and I put
a letter in with them: "Dear Parent—Your son/daughter
will be asked to complete a questionnaire on teen issues.
S/he will not be required to participate. Call me by _____
if you have any questions regarding this survey." I had no
response whatever, and almost all the students completed
the survey. A few stopped when they got to the part about
sex, and that was okay.

We repeated the questionnaire two years later.

The results of the survey didn't shock us, but it did the
parents. One item of special interest to parents was,
"Where did you get most of your basic sex information?"

"Friends," the majority answered.

"Where would you most prefer to get sex
information?"

"From our parents."

All through the years we've been trying to get the
parents to open up the lines of communication with their
kids. We give parent workshops, and we have pretty good
participation through the sixth grade, but after that, not
many parents come out.

A minority of people suggest that school-based clinics
take away the rights of parents, but we found that parents
were solidly behind us. We've been attacked, but always
by out-of-county people. I deal with these people by
saying, "What we're doing here is working. What is your
answer to teen pregnancy?" They don't ever have an
answer.

Clinic Develops from Student Needs

In **Jackson, Mississippi,** the **Jackson-Hinds Health Center**
also grew out of a concern for students' general health. "We'd
been doing sports exams, and we'd find problems such as
hypertension, undiagnosed kidney infections, diabetes—and
these were our athletes. We began to wonder about the health of
our other students," Aaron Shirley, Director, reminisced.

"Services were free at the parent clinic in Jackson, but teenagers didn't use them. Of about sixteen thousand patients at that time, less than seven hundred were adolescents, and we knew there were more out there."

---

*"Family planning is a natural part
of any doctor's office,
and that's the way we approached it."*

In 1979, the school-based clinic, funded through the United States Public Health Service, provided the personnel and the school provided the space. Within six months, they realized the severity of the teen pregnancy problem.

Ninety-four of the 550 girls in the school were pregnant. Clinic personnel started working with them, providing prenatal care and encouraging them to stay in school, "kind of holding their hands through it," Shirley commented. "Then we started our regular sessions of health education, and this is where we stress the need for prevention of teen pregnancy."

Parents have been supportive since the beginning, according to Dr. Shirley. He explained:

> *First we went to the PTSA, and they gave us their blessing. Once we got permission from the parents, the school officials were supportive.*
>
> *These kids had ringworm, chronic ear infections, all kinds of problems. We offered family planning services. Family planning is a natural part of any doctor's office, and that's the way we approached it. Parents give blanket approval for services.*
>
> *In that first school, which also has a day care center, the pregnancy rate has been cut about half, and the repeat pregnancy rate is way down. When we fail at prevention, at least we have healthy babies and the kids don't drop out of school. Recently one of our student mothers graduated from nursing school, two others from college, and several from junior college.*

When people oppose SBCs, we can remind them we
need the clinic so we can get the most out of the students.
If the kid is not anemic, if his vision and hearing are okay,
he'll be a better student. It costs the community $2,400 for
every kid that repeats a grade. It's a good investment to
provide health care. Now we have clinics in three addi-
tional schools in Jackson and one in rural Hinds County.
Two of the clinics are in junior high schools and one is in
an elementary school.

I've told them high school is too late. Now I'm concen-
trating on the elementary school. It opened this fall in a
very tough neighborhood in a school with six hundred
students. For the first time, we have a school that's
allowing us to serve preschoolers in students' families.

Board Mandates School-Based Clinics

Jackie Goldberg and Roberta Weintraub, members of the **Los
Angeles Unified School District Board of Education**, were
concerned about the rising pregnancy rate among junior high
and elementary schools in their district. They had heard about
school-based health clinics, and asked their staff to get some
statistics on students' health needs.

"We were staggered. Not only was there lots of pregnancy,
but all kinds of health problems not related to sex—heart
murmurs, diabetes, tumors, lack of inoculations. We said, 'Let's
go for it (SBC),'" Goldberg recalled.

Maria Reza, now a principal at San Fernando Junior High
School, was assigned in 1986 to the position of starting a school-
based clinic in the Los Angeles Unified School District. Three
years later the school district had three fully functioning SBCs.
The district provides the space and the administrators while
services are paid through private funding with some help from
the Public Health Department.

Reza remembers knowing nothing about SBCs when she was
assigned to the task of starting one. She attended an SBC
training session at the SBC Support Center in Houston, Texas,
and by that time a school nurse, Pam Wagner, was assigned to
assist her. Reza said:

Ours was so different because usually SBCs start from the ground up with a community group seeing the need and going to the school board. We had a mandate from the Board of Education, so we had to sell the community on the idea as we worked toward implementing the mandate.

"Now that we have the clinics, we'd have a big hue and cry if we ever closed them."

We immediately set up a community advisory committee, one for the whole district plus one for each school with a clinic. At one school we had the demonstrations and the marches—people from an out-of-county town felt we were going to hell on a fast boat to China, and that we were usurping traditional family values.

Well, that's the school with more sign-ups now than at the other sites, because families there are so poor, some aren't legal, and they have no other source of health care. They don't have to produce an immigration card with us. They just have to be students in the school. Seven hundred students signed up in our second year of operation.

Actually we haven't heard a word from the opponents since we opened. I think they thought they would stop the opening. Now that we have the clinics, we'd have a big hue and cry if we ever closed them. The word has spread that they help kids. They're the best testimony for themselves.

Goldberg discussed the two major controversial issues, the parent permission slip and the dispensing of contraceptives:

I wanted a blanket permission slip, but I was wrong. I was voted down, and it's worked. Almost nobody who uses the clinic specifies exceptions. The greatest exclusions are those who don't believe in blood transfusions. The fact that you can exclude certain services is a great selling point. I was wrong on that one.

*But on the dispensing of contraceptives, I was right. I
know kids will be kids, and I wanted contraceptives
available on campus. At one school the prescription is
written at the clinic, and they go across the street to the
pharmacist to have it filled. At another school, the
contraceptives are dispensed in the clinic.*

*I'm certain we'd have the same flack if we didn't
dispense contraceptives. If you're going to do a clinic,
you'll get some flack. The people who don't want them
think if you talk about it, the kids will have sex. Other
people who don't want clinics can't accept the fact that
they can't control everything their children do, and they
don't want to be reminded of that. Overall, parents have
been very accepting. So have the kids, and so have the
teachers.*

Concern for Restrictive Policies

In **Portland, Oregon,** the Multnomah County Department
of Human Services operates four school-based teen health
centers. The **Roosevelt Teen Health Center** opened in Feb-
ruary, 1986, and clinics at three other high schools opened a
year later.

Sue Imbrie, Coordinator of the Roosevelt clinic, worries
about diluting the services of SBCs. She commented:

*I've been concerned about the decrease in SBCs
offering birth control. I think people feel backing away
from controversy might help get rid of the flack, but
generally if the opposition wins that, they go after the
exams, then education, everything. Some have been quoted
as saying that's what they're after.*

*We need to recognize that there will always be people
opposed to contraceptive services for young people,
opposition based on dogma and not scientific fact. Which
do people think public policy should be based on—dogma
or scientific fact?*

*They aren't going to stop having sex because you have
these restrictive policies. I think it boils down to "Do you*

*really want to have any impact?" I think when we have a
non-voting, non-taxable age group, we have one of the
least powerful groups in the country.*

Imbrie would like to see clinics in elementary and junior high
schools, and she'd like services to be available to all young
people in the area, not limited to those currently attending
school.

Tactics for Dealing with Controversy

Constancia Warren, who had worked with the Board of
Education in New York City, came to the **Center for Public
Advocacy Research** the day public controversy about school-
based health clinics hit the front pages of the *New York Times*.
"A colleague told us, 'Controversy is actually an ally in disguise
here. Work with it. You have people in favor of SBCs who will
speak out now because they don't want the opposition to win,'"
she reported, then explained:

*The New York Board put a six-month moratorium on
distributing contraceptives, but all other clinic services
were continued. They also commissioned an independent
assessment of the clinic program. Those six months gave
us a chance to pull the facts together.*

*We learned that kids don't have access to health care.
We learned that only twenty percent of clinic visits deal
with reproductive health care. We also learned that
ninety-two percent of the parents that were interviewed
wanted abstinence counseling, eighty-five percent wanted
family planning counseling, and sixty-one percent wanted
either prescriptions written or distribution of contraceptives on campus. This helped the Board of Education
decide to support clinics. The outcry had been that the
clinics weren't wanted by parents and community, but this
showed that parents thought the clinics were doing a
terrific job.*

*The day after the school board voted to continue the
clinic program, people from all over the country called*

*clinic providers to congratulate us on our victory. We
proved that the opposition doesn't always have to win.*

Warren pointed out the importance of school-based clinics
being connected to a health care facility, somewhere students
can go when school is closed, or for care not provided by the
clinic:

> *You have to start with the parents, the school, and a
> provider who is interested. Sometimes a provider is
> interested, but there is no school nearby. Even more
> frustrating is when a school in a high-need area can't find
> a provider.*
>
> *Beyond providing badly needed health services, clinic
> providers tend to be caring adults who have non-
> judgmental attitudes toward kids. They aren't teachers
> who are grading them, and they aren't parents who might
> withdraw their love. They offer the kind of relationship
> kids may have had in the past with Scouts or adult leaders
> of other activities. Kids have a tendency to hang out in the
> clinic sometimes because they see it as a safe harbor.*

For those wondering about starting a school-based clinic,
Warren suggested contacting the Center for Population Options.
She recommends CPO's *Planning and Implementation Guide.*

Teens Offer Challenge

Rozanne was born four years ago when Val was thirteen.
Because of the child care and other special services at her high
school, Val will graduate from high school next semester. Val
was asked, "Did you want to get pregnant at thirteen?" She
replied:

> *No. I was having sex at twelve, and somebody should
> have told me, "Planned Parenthood is here. This is where
> you can get the protection." I didn't even know about it.*
>
> *I was a sixth grader learning about menstrual periods.
> When I was a sophomore, my baby was already two years*

*old, and that's when they started teaching us about STDs.
I can't remember being in health class and learning about
the pill or the IUD or anything like that.*

*I don't think they do a good job teaching you about
your own sexuality. It's like they expect you just to say
"No." When you get to age twelve or thirteen, you start
getting interested in the opposite sex. If it could be
brought out in the open and talked about, kids would feel
a lot less pressure to do it.*

*So many parents try to cover all this up too. They think
if you talk about it, you're going to do it. I think parents,
when a kid starts asking questions, should be honest and
not beat around the bush. If you're open and honest from
the beginning, perhaps your kid will come to you when
s/he needs birth control.*

*The reason I looked for sex was because I needed
attention and I needed love, and I thought that was love at
the time. It was a grown-up thing to do, and I thought it
could bring me love. Obviously it didn't.*

Working with sexually active teens offers many challenges.
We must continue to support sexual abstinence for adolescents
in every caring way we can, in our homes, our churches, our
communities, and our schools. We must help young people
develop high self-esteem and reachable goals so that they are
more likely to delay sexual intercourse until they are ready to
handle the responsibilities that go along with saying "Yes."

At the same time, we can't ignore the large numbers of teens
already sexually active. If we care about our youth and their
future, we will help them cope with the heavy responsibilities
they are assuming. Instead of putting obstacles in their way,
obstacles to receiving the good health care and the supportive
counseling they all need and deserve, we need to implement
programs to help them achieve satisfying lives.

CHAPTER 5

Considering Alternatives

The adolescent pregnancy prevention continuum does not stop with prevention of pregnancy. Many teenagers today, more than a million annually, are getting pregnant, and many of their partners are also teenagers.

A pregnant teenager has four legal alternatives. She may terminate her pregnancy, she may make and carry out an adoption plan for her child, she and her partner may marry, or she may become a single mother. About fourteen percent of teenage women's pregnancies end in miscarriage. Slightly less than half of the others have an abortion. About four percent carry out an adoption plan. Of those remaining, only thirty-nine percent get married. The others, whether for a short or long period of time, become single mothers.

The Marriage Alternative

The proportion of teen births occurring outside of marriage has quadrupled since 1960, from fifteen percent to sixty-one percent. Among black teen women, ninety percent are single at delivery. The percentage is forty-nine percent for white teen women.

---

*There is no easy alternative
in too-early pregnancy.*

We would like to believe that marriage would solve the problem of too-early pregnancy. However appropriate shotgun weddings may have seemed in the past, we know teens who marry because of pregnancy now are not likely to be married long. A cynic remarked, "Teenage marriage is a *temporary* cure for single parenthood."

Some teen marriages succeed. If a young couple decides to marry, they probably will need as much support as they would if they remained single. Both need to complete their education and obtain job skills. Prenatal care is as important to a married teenager as it would be if she remained single. The young couple may need help with child care. The needs continue, whether or not they marry.

Occasionally people still refer to special programs for teen parents as programs for *unwed mothers*. To exclude married teenagers from special services often means excluding young people in great need of support.

Alternatives counseling certainly includes an examination of the pros and cons of marriage as well as the other alternatives. But marriage is no quick fix for adolescent pregnancy.

No Quick Fix in Too-Early Pregnancy

There is no easy alternative in too-early pregnancy. Whether the teenager chooses abortion, adoption, single parenting, or marriage, she/they may never be the same again. Whatever the outcome of the pregnancy, support is needed for the person(s) involved.

Real crisis pregnancy counseling needs to focus on the needs of the woman and, if he's involved, her partner. It's not a place to indoctrinate already distraught women with one's own convictions.

We need to acknowledge our personal biases, then go on from there. Some people truly believe, for example, that adoption is a terrible thing, something no caring mother could ever do. A few teenagers have said, "Adoption is worse for the baby than abortion." That's their reality.

Others feel adoption is the solution to teenage pregnancy. "With all those lovely families wanting babies, why don't 'they' release?" they ask.

We cannot make
others' decisions.

While each of these opinions can be real and human and honest, neither should be foisted on someone else as she/they confront a complex, wrenching, life-altering decision. Each of us working with women or couples facing untimely pregnancy must honestly realize we don't ever have the answer for someone else.

We can help them look at all of their legal alternatives, point out some of the realities they may face with each choice, and support them as they make the decision. This must be done deliberately, patiently, and involve all the significant others who may be applying pressure on the decision-making. *We cannot make others' decisions.*

Each year about forty-six percent of all pregnant teenagers in the United States choose to have an abortion. For most, this is a difficult decision. For young women and their partners, sensitive and caring counseling is important both before and after abortion.

Before the abortion, she/they need to be assisted in looking at their alternatives. Why is she considering termination of her pregnancy? According to research, if she has an abortion because she thinks her parents or her partner give her no other choice, she is likely to regret the decision.

If she has always had strong beliefs against abortion, but thinks she now has no other choice, she may need extra help in looking at her choices, and in long-term counseling if she follows through with the abortion.

If, as service providers, our religious or moral system or our personal convictions do not allow us to provide this help, we need to refer her to someone else who can offer more unbiased assistance.

Counseling Technique Described

Lynn Leight, Founder and Director of the SHE (Sex, Health, Education) Center, Miami, Florida, has worked with hundreds of teens in her thirty-year career as a nurse, sex educator, and counselor. She has established the counseling program for the seventeen SHE centers across the United States. Abortions are not performed at the SHE centers, but a range of gynecological services, sexuality counseling, and parent seminars are offered.

Leight talked about the challenge in counseling pregnant adolescents:

> *Making a decision concerning an unplanned pregnancy is extremely difficult for adolescents. They tend to be fragmented because they're trying to please so many people, and they're bombarded with conflicting messages and confusing choices. They're disappointed that, even though they feel invincible on many levels, this has happened to them. They feel overwhelmed and powerless.*

At this point the most important thing is to create a bond of trust, and to diffuse the teen's anxiety, Leight pointed out. She often introduces open-ended questions which inspire role playing as the dialogue proceeds:

> *I ask, "Who else knows about your pregnancy?"*
> *If no one knows about it, I ask, "What do you think will happen if you tell your parents about your dilemma?"*
> *Her immediate response usually is, "They'll kill me."*
> *I then paradoxically agree with her. "You're right, they probably will kill you." She's likely to look at me, puzzled, and she may even laugh.*
> *Then I query, "The one thing I'm not sure about is, how will they kill you?" She's likely to smile a little.*

"Do you think they'll use a gun?" I ask, rather seriously. A bigger smile.

"Perhaps a knife?" I suggest. Then, "Oh, but I guess that would be messy. Do you suppose they'll slowly poison your food?" We both are now smiling and she's ready to talk about her realities.

"Do you think it's realistic to believe they'll kill you? How may they really respond? What kinds of feelings will they have?"

There's a sense of understanding that of course her parents won't kill her, and she may say they'll feel "disappointed," "angry," "hurt," or maybe even " violent."

If "violent" is her response, she's presented a red flag. I then ask, "Tell me about the last time your parents acted in a way you'd describe as violent." Now I must really focus in on her lifestyle.

Next I'll ask, "Tell me about the last time you told your parents something which really disappointed them. What happened?" This sets a framework as to how her parents react in other situations that may or may not be as dramatic as this. With this particular client, we may need to identify another trusted person in her life to whom she can turn at this time, perhaps an older sister, an aunt or uncle, a grandparent.

"Most of these young people
want to involve their parents,
but they're too frightened."

For the teen with the askable parent, but who is also fearful of sharing her news, I will role play, helping her first to determine the right time and place to discuss her situation with her parents.

She might not know the best time, so I give her some suggestions. We may narrow it down to a time when the identified person is likely to be most mellow and most accessible, perhaps in the evening before the TV goes on. Then I assume the role of the parent. She rehearses with

*me the way in which she will share the news, and I rebut
in the way that most simulates her parents' probable
response.*

*I believe most of these young people want to involve
their parents, but they're too frightened. The issue of
losing a parent's love is so paramount that they often feel
hopeless, almost paralyzed with fear. I believe that once
the teen sits down with a counselor who has the time, the
energy, and the compassion to walk through this trauma
with her, she is likely to gain the faith and confidence to
consult her parents, usually her most loving allies.*

*I find that these young women, even those who say
"Never, never never can I tell my parents. They'd kill me"
find that their parents do come through for them. After the
adult gets rid of the anger—which is often disappointment
in themselves for not recognizing their daughter's
vulnerability—the anger is displaced with support.*

*I provide the same dignity for all of the choices avail-
able. If we don't dignify each choice, we ultimately are
channelling each individual into a decision we believe is
right for her, and we don't have that right.*

Phyllis Elimeleck, Director, **Lady's Center, North Miami,
Florida,** provides alternatives counseling for pregnant teens.
She stressed the importance of thorough counseling before the
teen makes a decision. If she chooses to terminate the pregnancy, follow-up counseling is offered. Elimeleck stressed:

*Primary in our counseling is never to make the deci-
sion for them, never, never for anybody. We'll counsel
concerning all their legal options, and offer pros and cons
of each choice in as non-judgmental a way as possible, yet
totally supportive. We get the message across that we're
going to help her/them in any way we can.*

*We have to be supportive, as comforting as possible to
help her through a difficult time. At this point we never
ask, "Why weren't you more careful?" She already feels
terrible. We encourage the young ones to share their*

decision with a parent or a sister, someone they feel they can trust. I say, "Your mother might surprise you. She might turn out to be your best friend."

Many times this happens, and she'll tell me, "I never dreamed she would ever be supportive, but you were right."

If she considers termination of the pregnancy, we counsel very fully about the procedure from the beginning to the end. If she's continuing her pregnancy, of course we refer her to prenatal care.

If she terminates, we want her back for her three-week check-up. At that point, we help her go over her feelings, and we assist her in separating her feelings from those of others. We also emphasize her need for birth control at this time.

Concern for Mother and Child

Judy Peterson, Director of **BETA,** a comprehensive program for pregnant and parenting teens in **Orlando, Florida,** has a bias against abortion. She could speak quite strongly about the issue. In her counseling, however, she focuses on both the mother and baby:

We feel strongly that two lives are involved in a pregnancy, and we aren't doing our job unless both lives develop in a positive manner. Our job in talking with a woman facing a difficult pregnancy is to give her a little space to get in touch with what she feels, what she wants, what her dreams are.

"We don't look at the baby as the problem. The baby is a symptom of what's going on."

We help her define why she is doing what she's doing. Why is she continuing the pregnancy? Or why is she choosing to abort? Most women abort not because they want to have an abortion, but because they feel they have no other choice.

We have to be careful to protect the woman's right to continue her pregnancy as well as her right to abort. We give her choices. We look at other things that might help her solve her problem.

Is she looking at abortion because she feels if she doesn't abort her baby, she won't have a place to live? If that's her only reason, we can help her find housing. Or does she need health care? Does she need counseling? What are her needs? We give her a choice of services so she isn't aborting simply to solve a problem. We offer other ways of looking at the problem if she chooses to do so.

"We can't walk away and allow a perfect newborn baby to start losing ground almost immediately."

If she continues her pregnancy, we would like her to look at other programs as her baby develops—school, perhaps intensive counseling, certainly good health care. We don't look at the baby as the problem. The baby is a symptom of what's going on. If we simply help her abort or deliver without addressing what brought her to this point, we really haven't done our job.

Instead, we need to look at what these women and children need to be whole and healthy and happy. What brings peace and hope into their lives? That's where programs should start. Before you ever start developing a program, you ask yourself these questions.

Also involved in alternatives counseling, according to Peterson, is concern for the child after birth:

That's a big question because we know that children born to teen moms lag in cognitive development and communication skills. And that's not tolerable. We can't walk away and allow a perfect newborn baby to start losing ground almost immediately.

BETA's Breaking the Cycle program is designed to help defeat this projected negative outcome. (See Chapter Ten.)

Training for Foster Parents of Pregnant Teens

Some Crisis Pregnancy Centers provide "shepherding" or foster homes for pregnant teenagers. Sr. Maureen Joyce, Director of **Community Maternity Services, Albany, New York,** operates a group maternity home and other pregnancy prevention and care services. She also trains families to host pregnant teens. She discussed the need for such training:

> *If you're going to find foster or "shepherding" families, you have to be there to provide long-term training and education for the families. Some have young children and have never parented adolescents. If she doesn't meet her curfew, what do you do? How do you handle her boyfriend? If the family is out there on their own, you're likely to lose them when these crises come up. If you have someone with the family and the young mother, someone who may help them set up a kind of contract, it's more likely to work. It takes hard work, not only for the family, but also for the helping professional.*

"We're talking about a girl who has faced all kinds of things this family has never seen."

> *Our foster families go through a five-session training which deals with adolescent development, adolescent parenting and adoption, and other issues. Some families tend to get so involved that if she considers adoption, they don't support her decision. They tell her they'll keep the child until she's ready, or they know somebody who will take it. But they have to be objective. They can't be pressuring her.*
>
> *It's also the responsibility of the agency to say to the family, "If it doesn't work out, we're here to make a*

*change." We don't want a situation to be so difficult that
no one is prospering.*

*Sometimes people ask me to talk to groups about
setting up homes for pregnant teens. Often they think
we're talking about the sixteen-year-old all-American girl
who is very docile. But we're talking about a girl who has
faced all kinds of things this family has never seen. You
can't assume she has had the kind of nurturing you'd like
a sixteen-year-old to have. Yet some groups provide no
screening and no training for shepherding home
applicants.*

If you're involved in a foster home program for pregnant
teenagers, you'll need to offer counseling and in-service training
for prospective host families. It's not fair to expect families to
offer this service without professional assistance.

Making an Adoption Plan

Less than five percent of pregnant teenagers carry out adoption plans for their children, and many of the ninety-five percent
planning to parent are quite outspoken about their objections to
this alternative. Nevertheless, adoption needs to be supported as
one of the loving and caring options open to anyone involved in
a problem pregnancy.

The state of **Wisconsin** has funded the **Adoption Information Center** since 1986. This center was established by the
legislature to provide information about adoption to adolescents
and older women experiencing unplanned pregnancies. Their
goal, according to Lori Obluck, Project Coordinator, is to
increase public awareness of adoption as an alternative. Information and referral services are provided, and the Center also
offers training for professionals who work with adolescents and
young adults.

The Center also prepares Public Service Announcements for
radio and television, and has created several posters dealing with
adoption. Obluck says the Center receives about two hundred
calls per month from birthparents, prospective adoptive parents,
and professionals. Obluck exhibits adoption materials at

conferences, and frequently is responsible for workshops dealing with the topic.

Pregnancy alternatives counseling is a specialized area which demands knowledge of local and state laws and extensive training in decision-making and dealing with people in crisis.

Catherine Monserrat, adoption specialist and co-author of *Adoption Awareness: A Guide for Teachers, Counselors, Nurses and Caring Others* (1989: Morning Glory Press) stresses the importance of having decision-making groups and support groups after the baby is placed with the adoptive family:

> *Counseling is never **never** counseling them to relin-*
> *quish. People ask me, "How can I get them to place their*
> *children since all these wonderful people want to adopt*
> *babies?" I believe firmly that she should **never** be talked*
> *into releasing because somebody else wants a baby. She*
> *wants her baby too—adoption plans are seldom made*
> *because the mother doesn't want her baby. A mother*
> *makes an adoption plan because she decides that's the*
> *best decision for her child and, hopefully, for herself.*
>
> *Sometimes choosing and meeting the adoptive couple*
> *before delivery helps her finalize her decision because she*
> *can be more peaceful knowing she chose a good family for*
> *her child. Our job is not to convince her she should*
> *release. It's to help her make a decision with which she*
> *can live the rest of her life.*
>
> *I think it is our responsibility, when we work with*
> *pregnant teens, to provide an atmosphere that educates*
> *about and is supportive of all the alternatives. We need to*
> *display in our offices and on our walls posters and*
> *literature which support adoption as a positive choice.*
>
> *Staff attitudes filter to the young women very quickly. If*
> *staff members don't approve of all the alternatives, their*
> *attitudes and biases can affect their clients. It is essential*
> *that we work with staff and discuss these issues. Then, as*
> *a unit, we can decide which alternatives will be addressed*
> *and supported in our programs.*
>
> *Sound decisions are made from choices.*

Counseling Is Difficult Task

Teenagers facing too-early pregnancy must make perhaps the most difficult decision they have ever made or will ever make again. Each alternative needs to be weighed with extreme care. All possible accurate data must be presented by the counselor. At all times the welfare of all principals involved, the client cluster, must be considered.

Programs offering sensitive counseling and support services at this time are a crucial part of adolescent pregnancy prevention and care services.

Alternatives counseling is a difficult task. A young woman who is pregnant too soon is extremely vulnerable. She and her partner need caring support and assistance with decision-making perhaps more now than they ever will at any other time in their lives.

CHAPTER 6

Focusing
On Males

The adolescent pregnancy prevention continuum, of course, applies to young men as well as young women. Most of the pregnancy prevention programs and some of the teen parent services described in these books are designed for both males and females. We have never meant to suggest that pregnancy prevention and care services are or should be designed for one sex only.

Most often, however, these are services that focus primarily on young women. Young men may be welcome, but if the service is designed to attract young women only, the men aren't likely to participate. Reality suggests, therefore, that we look at some specific programs for males.

More Research on Females

Research on adolescent sexuality focuses primarily on adolescent females. Only a fraction of the money spent on birth control research is used for developing new male contraceptives. The research on adolescent sexuality concentrates primarily on females' sexual knowledge, attitudes, and behavior.

Research available on male sexuality issues suggest that teenage boys tend to be less informed about sexuality than are teenage girls. Part of the reason for this phenomenon may be that teenage boys, because of their need to seem macho, are less likely to ask their parents or teachers questions about sex. Also, most sex education occurring within families is done by the mothers, not the fathers.

Coupled with lack of accurate information are the sexist attitudes within much of our society. Boys are encouraged to have early sexual experiences while girls are supposed to say "No" to sex. One study found that, although seventy percent of the fathers surveyed wanted their sons to feel that premarital sex is acceptable, only two percent had ever mentioned contraception to their sons.

The media offers little positive modeling on sexual responsibility. Study after study reports that friends are a primary source of sexual information for both male and female teenagers. Some studies suggest that young males' reliance on friends for sexual information is higher than that of young females.

Among many teenage couples, the young man's attitude has a powerful influence on the couple's decision to use or not to use birth control. If most of his information and attitudes toward sexuality come from friends and the media, his education in these issues may be woefully lacking.

Why Male Involvement?

Wayne Pawlowski, Director of Training, **Planned Parenthood of Metropolitan Washington, DC,** suggests that one of our biggest problems is that nobody, including young men, know what we mean when we talk about male involvement and male responsibility:

> *When we say we want them to be more involved as contraceptors and more involved in the pregnancy, what do we mean? When you ask people how they feel about a*

male who doesn't like to use condoms so he carries sponges with him, half will say he's acting responsibly, and the other half will say he's not.

"If we define involvement only as child support, he doesn't benefit, he only suffers."

If she's pregnant and he has money, the kind of involvement and support we want from him is fairly clear— money. If he doesn't have anything, what we want gets fuzzy. Our message really is, "Be involved and responsible, but don't decide what that means until after she decides what she's going to do. Then we'll tell you how you can be involved and responsible." This leaves young men in an unclear position, and encourages them to opt out rather than to stay involved.

Sometimes it seems we have to trade her needs against his needs. If we define involvement only as child support, he doesn't benefit, he only suffers. What we wind up doing is pitting his suffering against her suffering. Then we say, "Why shouldn't he suffer? She does." It's okay for us to do this, but if we pretend it's something good for him when it's actually punitive, we're kidding ourselves and undermining our purpose.

In some states the paternity laws are extremely clear. In some states if you father a child when you're a teenager and you have no money, you don't have to contribute to child support as a teen. But as soon as you have something, the state will attach it. This may be punitive, but it's clear and males know exactly where they stand. I think this is okay, although it might be better to be more positive, and help them take responsibility up front.

Another important factor is the underlying hostility against men that exists in family planning. It tends to show up as soon as you start talking about male involvement. Many women who work in family planning have become angry at men for the situations in which they've left women, and rightfully so, but unless we can deal with that anger, we aren't going to provide a welcoming environment for men.

Teens account for only about one-third of the unintended pregnancies in the United States each year. Yet when we talk about male involvement, we generally mean teen involvement. I suspect we do that because teens don't have very much political power. If we were talking about white males over forty, we'd have a very different issue.

We want young men to communicate, yet in the young male mind, communication and sensitivity are feminine characteristics, and being feminine is equated with being homosexual. That terrifies them. If a boy is labeled gay by his peer group, how can he prove he isn't? By making a baby. Our cultural phobia about homosexuality plays a big role in the teen pregnancy problem.

We also have a mixed message on condoms. We've been pitching condoms for years and years, but only since AIDS have we realized people need instruction on how to use them. Most family planning information is written for women. We somehow assume men will know how to use condoms without instructions.

Because of all these issues, Pawlowski sees a need for a change in the whole system of sexuality attitudes and training. He believes, for example, that a clinic can change its climate in order to make boys think it's okay to be there.

A clinic wishing to move in this direction must first truly decide they want to provide services for males, and spend time training the staff appropriately, "not the hard medical stuff, but rather help them get in touch with their own attitudes toward males, and how these attitudes may get in the way of providing services for men," Pawlowski said.

Another issue is that of limited resources. If you're running a program for teen mothers and your funding doesn't cover all the services you'd like to provide, do you dilute those services even further by budgeting a component for fathers? There is no easy answer.

Prevention Starts in Childhood

Prevention programs for males as well as females must start in childhood. The young man with high self-esteem who has positive goals for his life is less likely to become a father before he's ready.

Providing help in developing those goals among young men is an important aspect of pregnancy prevention. It is also important that he be encouraged to delay sexual activity, and, when he becomes sexually active, to be responsible in terms of contraception until he is ready to parent a child. This triangle of prevention support is crucial.

If he has goals, but becomes a father too soon, those goals may never materialize. If he drops out of school, can't get a job, and has no hope for his future, he is more likely to resort to "making babies" in order to prove his masculinity to his peers or to "be someone."

Chapters Two, Three, and Four include descriptions of prevention programs from preschool through adolescence, most of which are designed for both males and females. Some programs, however, focus specifically on boys.

Boys and Babies is an innovative program for pre-adolescent boys involved in youth activities at the **Presbyterian Church of the Palms, Sarasota, Florida**. Sharon Winkler, who initiated the program in 1982, says the idea was the culmination of several factors: her volunteer work with other sexuality education programs, her background as a home economics teacher, and the fact that her own son was at the age when he was becoming more and more interested in sex and human development.

When the church opened a full-time infant care center, the program was introduced as a babysitting class for boys with a human sexuality component.

The course is composed of three units in which the boys learn how to diaper, feed, bathe, dress, play with and talk to babies, how to care for babies before they're born, how fathers can be involved in prenatal care, and about the human reproductive process and human development.

Winkler observed:

It seems logical to move backward from first learning to take care of babies, then learning how important it is to take good care of babies even before they're born, then learning how babies get in the womb in the first place, and finally learning how babies grow up and become teen- agers and adults capable of having babies themselves.

This program gives young boys an opportunity to have hands-on experiences with babies. Class experiences and homework assignments give the parents and boys the chance to talk about topics that would otherwise be difficult to broach.

Communication Focus for Males

ManTalk, a pregnancy prevention program of the **Forsyth County Health Department, Winston-Salem, North Caro- lina,** provides ongoing support and information for teen males aged thirteen to nineteen.

The program works to promote positive lifestyles and good decision-making skills by involving the male partner and opening communication channels with young men in a support group setting.

While establishing positive social support systems for teen males and promoting responsible sexual behavior, ManTalk also works to provide skill training in areas such as career develop- ment, parenting, academic goal achievement, self-esteem building, and job marketing.

ManTalk has a strong volunteer component, with adult males serving as role models for the program. All volunteers are screened, then participate in two training sessions prior to their work with the teenagers.

After completing the training, volunteers serve as support group facilitators at ManTalk meetings. They share with teenage males their life experiences, choices, achievements, and ob- stacles to personal goals. They talk about how they overcame some of these obstacles.

This personal approach has allowed mentoring and role modeling to occur between the teens and the adult volunteers. Social and cultural activities are used to augment the program,

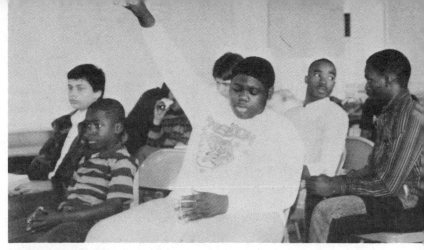

ManTalk group

and help develop closer trust-based relationships between volunteers and teens.

"While support groups are traditionally not seen as 'male activities,' they can be successful through the involvement of caring, non-judgmental adults who are willing to listen and share their experiences. It is also important to provide comprehensive programs which look not only at issues of responsible sexual decision-making, but also at issues such as employment, career planning, parent relations, sexism, racism, teen suicide, and substance abuse," commented Mary Grenz Jalloh, Director.

Beth Brandes, who founded TeenTalk (ManTalk's feminine counterpart) in Forsythe County, now leads Teen Up groups in the schools in Catawba County, North Carolina. Brandes pointed out the need for different kinds of discussions and activities in groups for early-adolescent boys or coed groups as compared to groups strictly for young women:

> *Boys find it much harder to talk about themselves. I encourage program providers to hang in there with boys' groups for more than six weeks, because at that point the boys are still talking about what macho studs they are. But that eventually breaks down, and then they'll talk about the important things in their lives including sexuality issues.*
>
> *I'm deeply saddened by the baggage young men have to carry. They tell me how upsetting it is to come home from a fight and have your dad say, "If you didn't win, I'll*

beat you up." Even when they try to change behavior, they have little support for it. I keep pointing out to them that it doesn't take a lot to make a baby, but the question is, is that baby going to be proud of you when he's fifteen? A lot of them can relate to that because their fathers were very young, and often were unable to support them emotionally or financially; they don't want to be like them.

Some families unconsciously promote their boys having sexual experience. Eighth grade boys tell me they don't "do it" with girls they like. The idea of using women is ingrained by the time they're twelve years old. They see women as objects. At twelve they're still malleable, though, and I'm finding our students are beginning to talk differently. I give them a lot of "what if" situations, trying to give them new ways to respond to things—"What would you do if an older guy messed with your little sister?" for example. They need that exercise in trying to determine what's right because society has said, "Go for it."

I'm suspicious of these interventions that happen three days a year in eighth grade, and they expect to change behavior. This can be a great springboard, but for high-risk kids, it's absolutely not enough. I point out to adult audiences that if your neighbor dies of a heart attack, you may eat better and exercise for about two weeks, but you have to have other reasons to sustain that change. Yet we're expecting kids to work out that to-be-or-not-to-be sexually active conflict through occasional presentations.

Male Involvement Programs from MOD

William R. Randolph, Deputy Director, Community Services Department, **National Office, March of Dimes Birth Defects Foundation (MOD),** notes that the interest which the adolescent male population has today in maternal and child health is greater than it has been in years, but stresses there still needs to be an increased awareness by males, particularly adolescent males, in the issues surrounding maternal and child health.

Randolph talked about a project in which thirteen males aged nineteen, categorized as working poor and/or receiving public assistance, were involved in focus groups designed to provide information about the needs of minority youths. The purpose of these focus groups was to get youths to articulate their ideas on maternal and child health issues and their role in adolescent pregnancy.

At first these young men talked about the importance of "scoring" sexually. Then they were asked how they would react if they impregnated somebody. Would they want that person to get good prenatal care? Would they encourage her to do so?

As the conversation continued, these young men expressed their concerns in these areas. "It's not the kind of information that is freely and immediately conveyed," Randolph commented. "You need some give and take before communication develops, and these interests surface."

Another **March of Dimes** project is the video, **"Clear Vision,"** a film in which a young man experiences pregnancy, morning sickness, and rejection from his partner. He worries about prenatal care and other situations typical of a pregnant teen's life. The film was created as a catalyst for discussion, preferably in groups of twenty-five to thirty teenage males. It helps young men express their feelings and their presumed responsibilities with these issues.

Project Alpha is another **March of Dimes** project, this one done in collaboration with Alpha Phi Alpha Fraternity, Inc. Project Alpha explores the problem of teenage pregnancy from the male perspective. In some areas, Project Alpha is a single session lasting from half a day to a three-day retreat. Other chapters sponsor several Project Alpha sessions each year.

The Project Alpha Leader's Guide, available from local March of Dimes chapters, provides a step-by-step approach to planning and conducting a program. Information about human reproduction and development and the psychosocial and legal consequences of teenage pregnancy gives participants a sound factual framework.

Participants are encouraged to clarify values, set goals, and make decisions consistent with their goals. The program urges young men to learn facts, understand responsibility, and share information with peers, family members, and their communities.

Health Enhancement for Boys

The Shiloh Baptist Church, Washington, DC, runs the **Male Youth Health Enhancement Project** in collaboration with the DC Department of Public Health. Boys aged nine to seventeen, about thirty each day, spend several hours after school at the Shiloh Family Life Center.

It is a comprehensive project which, according to director Andre Watson, assists young men in their transition from boyhood to manhood. Various activities point toward this goal: Rites of Passage and manhood training program, daily study hall, weekly workshops, field trips, athletic/recreation activities including football, basketball, ping-pong, "a menu of activities to implement our goal of assisting young men," Watson reported. He continued:

> *How do you find young men? You give them something they want. We want to prevent teen pregnancy, but we go beyond that because most guys still perceive pregnancy as a woman's problem. That's what society tells them.*
>
> *To get around that, we need activities that meet their interests. Most young guys need job training or employment. Health education for guys may not be strongly motivating, but once they're here, and we offer them the things they want, we can work on the health issues too.*
>
> *We need films and posters that appeal to males, that say, "You have a place here." We provide things they like, and use that as a buffer to get them to do the things we want them to do. We want them to study for an hour each day, so we put basketball after that hour of study. When we have a ski trip, he can go only if he has attended study hall a certain number of days.*
>
> *We have a conference each spring, and we combine it with a basketball tournament plus other sports tournaments. They have to go to the conference if they play in the tournament.*
>
> *Our after-school program starts with the study hall. They can't come in here after the study hour. Kids will come in at 4:30 p.m. with some kind of line, but unless his*

*mother calls and says he didn't come for a good reason,
we send him back home.*

*Attendance is a strong motivation for many of our
activities. We have to keep a lot of activities going because the minute one is over, if there's nothing else down
the road and he came because of the field trip, he won't
come back. We have to keep it hyped up.*

The program employs two full-time counselors who go into
the schools to talk with counselors and teachers. They monitor
clients' grades, and often find improvement after the boys have
participated in the project. "It took us a year to get them to come
to study hall," Watson added. "For many, this is the first time
they've been held accountable."

African American Project for Youth

Paul Hill, executive director, **East End Neighborhood
House, Cleveland, Ohio,** feels strongly that pregnancy prevention among African American youth is dependent on a restruc-
turing of male socialization. Working toward this objective, Hill
implemented a Rites of Passage program called **Simba
Wachanga** which is Kiswahili for young lions. He describes it
as a guidance system through which African Americans speak to
their young males.

The male focus of the program, he emphasizes, in no way
minimizes the importance of similar rituals for females. In fact,
a similar Rites of Passage for young women, Malaika, is part of
the **Simba/Malaika Network** sponsored by the East End Neighborhood House. These Rites of Passage are designed to provide
positive, culturally specific, and structured programs to help
youth progress from childhood to manhood/womanhood.

Young men participate in the Simba program at least a year,
two to four hours each week. Sex education is included in the
wide range of skill development areas provided to participants.

Positive male role models with a sense of their African
identity are integral to the program, Hill said. These men, known
as the Council of Elders, are instructors and Big Brothers
working under the direction of the program coordinator.

An important part of implementing a Simba project is identifying a sponsoring organization and recruiting a Council of
Elders who have the time, skills, commitment, interest, creativity, patience, and capacities to care and share, Hill said. The
coordinator is selected from this group.

Ideal sponsors are churches, fraternal and professional
organizations, and neighborhood community associations. The
Simba process can be adapted and used in school settings with
Cub and Boy Scouts, group homes, Boys Clubs, and other youth
groups. Parental involvement is an important part of the process.
"Creativity and flexibility in utilizing the model is essential, and
an understanding and knowledge of Afrocentricity is crucial,"
Hill concluded.

Males Often Stereotyped

Ed Pitt, former director, **Adolescent Male Responsibility
Program, Health and Environmental Services Department,
National Urban League,** talked about the stereotypes surrounding young males, especially African American inner-city
poor youth:

> *We're too quick to judge African American males as
> sexually irresponsible. The idea that the only badge of
> courage for the inner-city kid is to be a parent is a stere-
> otype and a myth. Almost none of the guys who are
> parents intentionally got a girl pregnant, or insisted that
> she not use contraception. Somehow we have the notion
> that these guys convince girls to have babies for them, and
> that they have sex with the intention of making a baby.
> That is the exception rather than the rule.*
>
> *Another myth is that, in addition to all these guys
> wanting to make babies, they completely shrug off their
> responsibility when the girl gets pregnant. That's not true,
> although many may not take the responsibility for rather
> complex reasons.*
>
> *First, many boys don't know about the pregnancy until
> late in the pregnancy or after the birth occurs. If they're
> told at birth, tremendous denial may set in.*

Another group of boys, when they hear about the pregnancy, insist on the girl getting an abortion. If she doesn't, the boy refuses to carry out his responsibility. He's the perfect example of someone who had no intention of parenting. But he didn't take the next step of either not having sex or using a condom.

"Men have somehow bought into the notion
that they can't say 'No'
when they think sex is expected."

You also have guys with the romantic notion of getting married, being a couple, and having a beautiful baby. We see a lot of guys who acknowledge paternity initially, and for awhile take pride in having parented.

"Okay, now you have this pretty baby, how are you going to provide for him?" That part was never figured out.

Finally, you have young fathers who are denied any real opportunity to parent by the mother's family. In these instances, it's not at all uncommon for the girl's parents to agree to assist her and her child as long as the girl remains out of contact with the young father.

I urge that we not go for the stereotypical picture of the male, especially the inner city African American male.

Pitt also talked about male expectations, and the changes occurring because of the threat of AIDS:

Men have somehow bought into the notion that they can't say "No" when they think sex is expected of them. They think they're expected to be sexually active, sexually knowledgeable, willing to perform. And until recently they usually weren't expected to take responsibility for prevention. So until the AIDS phenomenon, males have not been very prevention conscious in recent times.

Prior to AIDS, males tended to have a low regard for male contraception, but we're seeing real changes in the

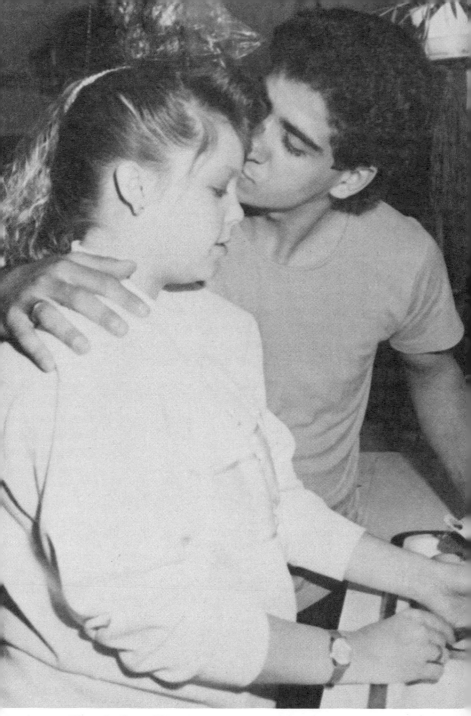

Photo by Joyce Young

*attitudes of sexually active youth today. We see them
accepting condoms to a much greater extent than they did
a few years ago. Community education and outreach
efforts from the health and education people are teaching
kids about the risks—from pregnancy to AIDS— of
unprotected sex.*

*When I speak with boys' groups, I ask them to show me
who has condoms in their pockets, and I'm surprised at
the number of boys who walk around now with condoms.
Five years ago that was not the case.*

*We know that with awareness will come behavior
change.*

The National Urban League operates a highly regarded multi-
media campaign with the theme, "Don't make a baby if you
can't be a father. Think before you do."

In addition to the media campaign, some fifty-five local
Urban Leagues operate male-focused prevention and service
programs. An example is **The Urban League of Albany Area,
Inc.**, which, in collaboration with the New York State Department of Labor, established the **Fatherhood Program**. This
program provides employability and life skills management
services to a population of unemployed, minority teenage
fathers.

The program focuses on parenting readiness, education, and
advocacy, plus job assessment, counseling, placement, and
follow-up. Average age of the participants is nineteen, and the
majority have never completed high school and were not
employed at the time they entered the Fatherhood Program.

Evaluation shows the majority made educational and/or
employment gains. Forty-five percent were employed while
twenty-nine percent enrolled in an education facility, either for
job training or to work toward a high school diploma.

An overwhelming majority of the participants felt services
provided by the program had helped them. Many reported a
positive relationship with their child(ren), with ninety-two
percent reporting contact at least once a week with their
offspring.

Support for Teen Males

Sally Brown, Director of the **Maine Young Fathers Project,** also feels young fathers are stereotyped as being uncaring. She commented:

> *Many times when he doesn't come forward, it's not because he doesn't care. It's because he's being excluded by the girl's family or by his own family encouraging him not to get involved. The social worker serving the young mother may also make him feel unwanted. We don't invite him in—then we notice he's absent, and we blame him.*
>
> *I realize there are young fathers who, because of physical abuse or other reasons, shouldn't be involved. As with other groups, however, we need to start by assuming he's okay and that he cares.*
>
> *We mustn't give up easily on him. Young fathers often take extra outreach, perhaps because men aren't used to asking for help. If we don't see him for a couple of weeks, we need to call him. He needs to know we haven't forgotten about him.*

Before moving to Portland, Maine, Brown was the Documentation Specialist for the Teen Age Parent Program (TAPP) Fatherhood Project, San Francisco, California. After being involved in TAPP's strong father support system, Brown found nothing similar in Maine. She decided the TAPP Fatherhood Project model would be useful in this primarily rural state.

She applied for and received a grant from the National Center on Child Abuse and Neglect on the premise that abandonment by fathers is a form of child neglect. The focus of the program is to keep fathers involved physically as well as financially with their children whether or not the relationship with the mother breaks off.

The father, whatever his age, is contacted by the Department of Social Services in Maine as soon as his impending fatherhood is known. He is asked to go in and discuss his obligations for the mother's prenatal care and for child support. Many young fathers, according to Brown, simply throw the paternity papers

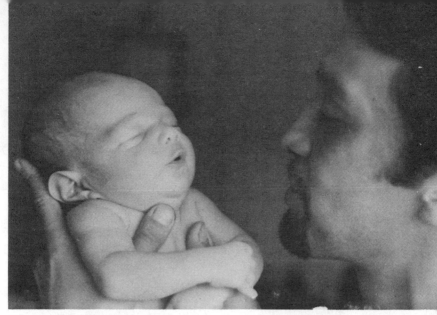
Photo by David Crawford

away. When that happens, the child support enforcement office takes the case to court.

If the father doesn't go to the court hearing, he'll be billed for the mother's prenatal and delivery expenses as well as for the full support of his child.

On the other hand, if he responds to the first request for an interview with the support officer, he may be able to have some of his obligations waived if necessary. Brown explained:

> *We're working with young fathers to bring them into the child support office and negotiate reasonable arrangements. We feel strongly that he needs to be financially responsible for his child, but it's not a good idea to drop out of school and get a job at McDonald's.*
>
> *The key is getting the father into the child support office to negotiate.*

The Young Fathers Project clients include men up to the age of twenty-four because, according to Brown, the majority of the fathers of children born to teenage women are in their early twenties. In fact, in California in 1986, only 28.3 percent of the 52,718 babies born to teenage women were fathered by men nineteen years old or younger, according to Claire D. Brindis.

(1988: *Adolescent Pregnancy and Parenting in California,*
page 32)

One Young Fathers Project client, Eric, twenty-year-old
father of Erin, two, and Brent, eight months, shared his story.
He and Regina were married while both were in high school.
They're separated now, and Eric is thinking of going into the
Army. Asked how he reacted to Regina's first pregnancy, he
responded, "Scared. I didn't believe it at first. It just happened,
and it's hard, real hard."

He recalls having no future plans when he was in high
school. He described himself as a "state child":

> *I was taken away from my mother when I was seven,
> and bounced around different places. Every time I got
> used to a family, I had to move. I've been in shelters,
> private schools, foster families, and it's a hard way to
> grow up. I've seen my mother twice since I've been on the
> state.*
>
> *We're trying to make our marriage work. Sometimes
> she wants it, sometimes she doesn't.*
>
> *I like the Young Fathers Group. It's fun to go to, and I
> usually bring one of my kids with me. I brought Erin with
> me today, and my son came along last week. We talk
> about lots of things—child abuse and how to handle it if
> one of your kids starts acting up. I've been doing better—
> using time-out instead of hitting.*

The project staff, in addition to Brown, consists of three case
managers, each working at one of the three project sites, plus
about thirty male volunteers. The case managers help the young
fathers obtain the services they need. "We don't focus just on
jobs," Brown said. "We also focus on positive parenting, nutrition education, childbirth education—the array of services we'd
provide for a young mother."

The male volunteers, called sponsors or mentors, are support
persons for the young fathers. They call or see their young
clients weekly, and follow up to see that the young men carry
through with their case plans.

"It's very important to have men involved, and not just a token male," Brown stressed. "It's not that women can't play a role, but to be effective, men must be involved in male support projects."

Teen Father Project

Teenage parent programs generally focus on the needs of young mothers, and involvement of the father is likely to have low priority. Some programs do, however, offer special groups for young fathers, and a few are admitting fathers into comprehensive school programs originally designed for school-age mothers.

The Teenage Parent Program (TAPP), Louisville, Kentucky, has an active fatherhood program. Young fathers, accompanied by babies and girl friends/wives meet weekly in a comfortable, apartment-like setting within the alternative school facility. They receive instruction in parenting, prenatal health, and family planning along with individual and group counseling. For couples who plan to share the delivery process, a coaching class is available once each school semester.

Education and employment are emphasized, and the fathers are strongly encouraged to continue in school and/or to obtain job skills through vocational programs.

Approximately 160 young fathers participate annually in the Fatherhood Program. An important feature of the program is the support provided by the young fathers for each other. The group provides an opportunity for young men to ventilate their feelings with their peers and receive guidance from group leaders.

School-age fathers can also enroll in the day program at TAPP, according to Georgia Chaffee, Principal:

> *Two young men enrolled in our school program. They applied themselves, they were interested in learning good parenting skills, and they came back to evening sessions with their wives. I made sure they understood this was not a place to hold hands as you walk down the hall. They understood that. In fact, they didn't have the same classes as their wives.*

Condoms Aren't Enough

Prevention for teenage men requires more than condoms and parenting education. For young teens, opportunities for recreation may be enough, but to older teens, getting a job is likely to be most important, and low wage, temporary, dead-end jobs won't suffice. Somehow, they must be offered training that will lead to at least the possibility of supporting their families.

Young men who have been on the streets may not be equipped for regular job market training. They need extensive services in drug rehabilitation, remedial education, and health services in addition to job training and parenting education.

The fact remains that young men need more information about sexuality than they get, and they need reasons not to get somebody pregnant—education and job opportunities and job training.

They, too, must have something to look forward to that says, "I don't want to have a baby at sixteen."

CHAPTER 7

Serving Pregnant Teens

We all want mothers to deliver healthy babies. We want teenagers to continue their education, make and carry out career plans, and be happy and productive citizens. Teenagers who are pregnant or parenting need special help to achieve these goals.

If you're planning services for pregnant teenagers, think as comprehensively as possible. The triad of education, social, and health services is essential for most pregnant adolescents. Babies born to teenage mothers are more likely to be born too small and too soon, and to have developmental problems. Babies of young teens are two to three times more likely to die in the first year than are those born to mothers in their twenties.

During pregnancy the young woman is more likely to be anemic or to suffer from pre-eclampsia than is her older and pregnant sister. Early and continuous prenatal care is extremely important for her. It is well documented that early intervention through education, a supportive family, and social, health, and nutrition services can significantly decrease these risks.

Need for Social Services

The pregnant teen's social service needs may be intense because of the emotional condition her pregnancy has produced or intensified. If she chooses to terminate her pregnancy, she needs to have caring and supportive counseling available. If she makes an adoption plan for her child, she needs the help of a capable, loving professional. If single parenthood or marriage is her choice, she is likely to need counseling help.

Whichever alternative she chooses, she may need financial help. She may need housing. She will always need someone who cares, who she can depend on to be there when needed.

A special kind of school program may also be desirable. Over and over, young women talk about the support they receive from each other when they're part of a group of pregnant students. "They know what I'm going through," they remark.

Although some very comprehensive programs have been developed for pregnant and parenting adolescents, certainly no one person, or even a single program needs to answer all of these special needs. Some programs and agencies, for example, focus on alternatives counseling. Whether it's a Crisis Pregnancy Center, a Planned Parenthood office, or an adoption agency, the program personnel probably won't offer a full-blown school program or complete health services. Instead, they will refer clients to other services as needed.

If She Miscarries

According to *Teenage Pregnancy: An Advocate's Guide to the Numbers* (1988: Children's Defense Fund), 13.4 percent of teen pregnancies end in miscarriage. The young woman experiencing a miscarriage may have mixed reactions. If the pregnancy was not welcomed, the miscarriage may appear to wipe out the problem. She may, however, grieve as older women do for the baby who will never be. She may feel guilty as she wonders if something she did or didn't do caused the miscarriage.

The teenager experiencing miscarriage needs caring support and counseling sensitive to her needs. She doesn't need to be reminded that her "problem" is gone. If she is in an on-going relationship, she may need family planning guidance and assistance in obtaining contraceptives. If she says she "won't ever do it again," respect her choice—but at the same time help her understand that if she changes her mind, whether deliberately or in a moment's passion, she needs to protect herself from another untimely pregnancy.

Promoting Prenatal Care

The **March of Dimes Birth Defects Foundation (MOD)** has been working for twenty-five years in the area of adolescent pregnancy. Anita Gallegos, Director of Community Services, Southern California MOD, explained:

> *The reason we became involved in adolescent pregnancy at the beginning was the poor outcome of pregnancy that teenagers were experiencing as they had babies before their own bodies were fully developed. We realized that being pregnant before age seventeen was a high-risk factor in pregnancy outcome.*
>
> *Now we offer information and referral because we want teenagers to find a place where they can go for prenatal care. Locally we're having a bus placard blitz in cooperation with the county. The bus company gave us free space on a thousand buses that run in the highest risk areas where statistics show the poorest outcome for pregnancy. We pay for putting up and taking down the signs. The placard says, "Do you need prenatal care? Call (phone number)."*
>
> *I was thrilled to learn about some research done in five sites across the country to see what kids knew about getting prenatal care. They were asked, "If you or your girlfriend were pregnant, would you know where to go?" A fifteen-year-old said, "I saw this number on the bus."*
>
> *We also worked with the Department of Health and other people to prepare free prenatal care information and make it available in five languages.*
>
> *We're encouraging the county to buy into the need for having a pregnancy referral number so people can find a place for prenatal care close to where they work or live.*

Teen Clinic Provides Comprehensive Care

Early prenatal health care for pregnant teenagers is essential,
yet most young teens get no prenatal care in the first trimester.
About one in five receives no care before the third trimester.

**American River Hospital Teen Clinic, Sacramento,
California,** provides comprehensive health care to pregnant
teens; well-baby care and immunization follow-up for their
infants; counseling and case management for pregnant and
parenting teens and their families; family planning services,
information and education for prevention of teen pregnancy and
AIDS, and screening and treatment of various adolescent health
concerns.

Funded with a variety of grants, the program shows amazing
outcomes for pregnant clients. Of 134 deliveries covered in the
1987-1988 Annual Report, only eight percent were Caesarean
deliveries compared to the national rate (for women of all ages)
of twenty percent. Only three babies (2.2 percent) weighed less
than 5 1/2 pounds, and average birthweight was seven pounds,
seven ounces. Fifteen percent of the teen mothers had episioto-
mies, and only twenty-seven percent received any medication in
labor. Ninety-nine percent of the babies had an Apgar score of
seven to ten at five minutes after delivery.

The Teen Clinic started when staff at the hospital noticed a
lot of teens coming in to deliver, and no special services were
available for them, according to Karen Dodge-Keys, Director of
the Teen Clinic:

> We felt the teenagers needed extra care because
> usually this was their first introduction to health services.
> Some hadn't even seen a doctor. They were walk-in
> patients. We felt these kids had no support system. What
> could we do about it?
>
> We put together a committee and wrote a Maternal
> Child Health grant to the state, and that was the grant that
> got us started. We decided to utilize a Certified Nurse
> Midwife because we thought this gave us a higher chance
> of having someone who would be compassionate and
> understanding toward the teenagers. We also hired a

*social worker and a registered dietitian so we could serve
our clients' psychosocial and nutrition as well as their
health needs. We hired a health educator to teach Lamaze
(childbirth preparation) and serve as a go-between to get
teens back to school if they have dropped out.*

*All of our patients deliver with the aid of a midwife at
the American River Hospital in Carmichael. If there is a
complication, an obstetrician comes in. Transportation is
a major problem, so we go in a van every week to two of
the teen parenting school programs and bring the girls
back for their health care.*

Routine psychosocial care plans include parenting education
regarding infant care, development, safety, and well-baby needs.
Additionally, the social worker assists patients in developing a
plan for support during labor and delivery, for help after the
birth, and facilitates patients having all necessary supplies ready
for the baby.

Psychosocial assessments and care plans may also pertain to
specific pregnancy-related issues, such as adjustment to pregnancy, young ages, adoption planning, or shared parenting.
Further, the social worker addresses educational goals, housing
stability, transportation access, and financial adequacy. Social
relationships with family, father of the baby, and friends are
evaluated in terms of the amount of support or stress provided,
as well as the past or present existence of physical, sexual, drug,
or alcohol abuse.

The social worker attempts to see high risk patients at each
clinic visit, moderate risk patients once monthly, and low risk
patients one time each trimester. All patients receive two postpartum social work visits.

Additionally, three case managers in the Adolescent Family
Life Program (AFLP) handle a total of eighty cases within
Sacramento County. The case managers meet with clients either
at their schools, homes, or at the Teen Clinic. Clients are seen,
according to their needs, on a regular basis.

School enrollment and attendance are top priorities, and considerable time and effort are spent working with the school

systems and special school programs to achieve these goals. Of the twenty-one school dropouts among the eighty clients, fourteen were re-enrolled in school.

Another example of a health clinic focusing on the needs of adolescent maternity patients is the **It's a New Life! Teen Pregnancy Program, Appleton, Wisconsin.** It's a New Life! is an eleven-week series which includes prenatal and Lamaze training plus twice-a-week prenatal exercise for pregnant teens. For those patients who have no one to coach them through labor and delivery, volunteer mentors are provided.

In addition, support groups for the partners and for the parents of the pregnant teens are scheduled twice during each series. The grandparent group provides resource and counseling support plus gives participants a chance to share their frustrations and lash out without making the teen the target, according to Carol Heid, Director. The fathers' sessions are led by a male counselor who helps the young men look at such issues as their roles and responsibilities, parenting, communication with their partners and families, and legal issues.

Prenatal Health Services at School

Some school programs for pregnant teens provide comprehensive health and social services on site. Caroline Gaston, principal, **New Futures School, Albuquerque, New Mexico,** described the intensive health services available for her students.

When the student first comes to New Futures, she sees a counselor and one of the four nurses on staff. The nurse does a health history and determines whether the young woman is receiving prenatal care. If she's not, which frequently happens, the nurse talks with her about her alternatives. She explains that the student can have her prenatal care at New Futures, and about half of the students agree to do so.

The University of New Mexico Medical School brings a prenatal care clinic to New Futures one day each week. They provide the staff and the school provides space. The clinic team includes an obstetrician, two nurse practitioners, a nutritionist, a family planning counselor, a laboratory technician, and a clerk. They do exams and simple lab work, all of which are free

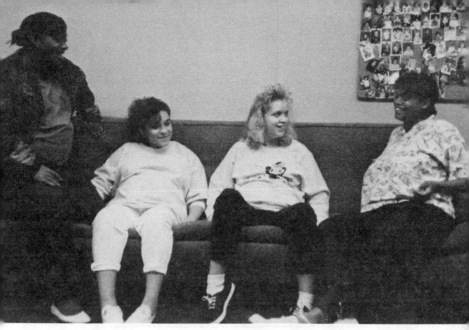

Photo by David Crawford

to any student at New Futures. Postpartum family planning services are also provided. If the student chooses to deliver at University Hospital, her fee is on a sliding scale according to her income.

According to Gaston, even students who have private insurance or qualify for Medicaid doctors may choose the school clinic for care. She talked about the advantages of on-site health care:

> *I think it's more effective health care because the clinic staff often meets with our nurses and sometimes our counselors after seeing the students. If there is a concern about someone's blood pressure, for example, our nurse can check it every morning. Receiving care here allows for continuity of care, and she misses fewer classes.*
>
> *The University of New Mexico also brings a family practice clinic here one day a week staffed by a resident. For that one, we provide the nurse, and we make the appointments. This is available to the babies as well as the students.*
>
> *The Public Health Department brings a well-child clinic for immunizations one day a month, and a Women,*

*Infants and Children Supplemental Nutrition (WIC) clinic
here weekly.*

*The important thing in working with teen parents is
that you're most effective if you're doing something* **with**
them rather than **to** *them. We help them assume the
responsibility for understanding what's happening to them
for self-care. Our eighteen-week daily health class makes
this possible.*

*One-to-one talks between a nurse and a student with a
sick baby on her lap are extemely effective learning
moments.*

*On-site clinics, the health classes, and individual
health counseling work together to promote the health of
our students and their children.*

"If we're in a school setting, we've got to be sure she's also getting the health services she needs."

---

*We also know that nutrition is an important part of the
health program. Our nurses do a nutrition history, a
three-day total recall, then a follow-up about how the
students might be able to make some changes.*

*They don't criticize what the girls are eating, but make
suggestions as to what they might be able to do, always
remembering that many don't have control over the food
served at home.*

*We were able to make minor changes in school
lunches, and we have a salad bar which the girls use a lot.
It's nice to see how, as the school year goes on, more and
more of our students are using that salad bar. We also
serve a fresh fruit snack every afternoon. Nutrition is
partly services and partly counseling and education.*

*Someone in another school program once told me they
were strictly an educational program. When I suggested
the girls should be getting prenatal care, it was a surprise
to her. This wasn't the school's responsibility, she said. I
didn't agree at all.*

In any setting we need to be sure this happens. If we're in a school setting, we've got to be sure she's getting the health services she needs.

Combining Services in Small Districts

Not many schools in the country offer the comprehensive services provided by New Futures. Many schools, in fact, have no special program for pregnant students. Even with careful attention to outreach, many small districts do not have enough pregnant students to merit a special teacher.

One program covering several school districts may be the answer. **New Horizons,** a school program designed for pregnant teens, is the result of cooperation among three rural school districts in **Texas**.

About fifty young women each year come from **Burleson, Crowley**, or **Joshua** school district. Enrollment opens every six weeks, and students may remain after delivery until the beginning of the next grading period.

New Horizons, Burlison, Texas

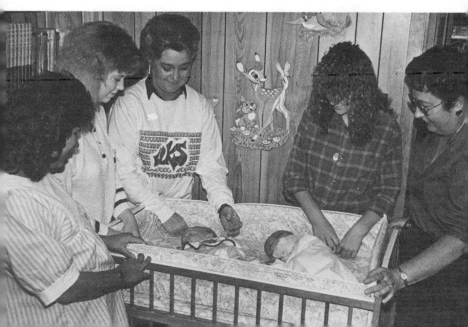

Mary Foster started New Horizons when, as a home teacher, she had eleven pregnant students at one time. She and another home teacher asked all the pregnant home study students to come in together, first just for one morning each week. The full-scale program evolved from there.

Under Foster's supervision, each student continues the academic classes she was taking at her home school. Frequent speakers from the community—nurses, Lamaze teacher, attorney, adoption counselor—offer their expertise to the students. Students return to class two weeks after delivery, and they may bring their babies with them.

Foster stressed the need for publicizing the program. Each winter she invites school board members, principals, superintendents, parents, and counselors from all three districts to a brunch at New Horizons. "I display students' work, and our guests know something good is happening here—especially after the parents talk about how much this has helped their daughter.

"You have to put more of yourself into a program like this, more than if it were just a job, or it won't succeed," Foster concluded.

Linking Social, Health, Education Services

Family Focus, Lawndale, Illinois, provides comprehensive social and health services at no charge to pregnant teens. Lawndale is an extremely low-income area of Chicago where about one thousand teenagers give birth each year. The Family Focus program, modeled after Our Place in Evanston, Illinois, was planned as an extension of a school-age pregnancy program at one of the high schools. Gilda Ferguson-Smith, Director, explained:

> *This area has a high school dropout rate and high infant mortality. Included in the proposal was job training, GED preparation, and a health component for pregnant teens. Through a grant with the local hospital, we pay for the prenatal care and delivery of the babies. All we ask is that she be involved with us for a full year if she gets the health service.*

*With our program she has a consistent doctor, consis-
tent care. A health educator nurse from the hospital helps
her set up her appointments and goes with her on the
appointments. This makes an incredible difference.*

*We also have weekly prenatal groups at the center with
a health component one week, and the next week, social
support. We make lots of home visits. We see, on the
average, about 110 expectant and parenting teens two
days each week.*

*We started this when we noticed the girls who were in
school during pregnancy weren't returning after the baby
was born. Support during the pregnancy and after delivery has made a lot of difference. Now the majority are
in school.*

Ferguson-Smith stressed that staff is the key to this kind
of program because their client families have so many
problems. They work closely with the extended families of
the pregnant and parenting teens and of the children in their
prevention program.

First they assess the family's individual needs, then put
together a family service plan including health, education,
and social service needs. Direct help and needed referrals are
built into the plan. A great many community resource people
are involved in the Center.

"We don't just open the doors and the girls come in and
have a good time. We must do so much more," Ferguson-
Smith mused.

Fairbanks Counseling and Adoption (FCA) works closely
with the **Fairbanks, Alaska,** Health Center, local Adolescent
Health Coalition, and the public schools to meet the needs of
pregnant and parenting teens, according to Cathy Mikitka,
coordinator of FCA pregnancy counseling.

FCA is a private, non-profit social service agency serving a
large geographic area of central Alaska. The program offers
various services and support groups for pregnant and parenting
teens including individual pregnancy counseling, pregnancy and
parenting support groups, foster homes, adoption services,

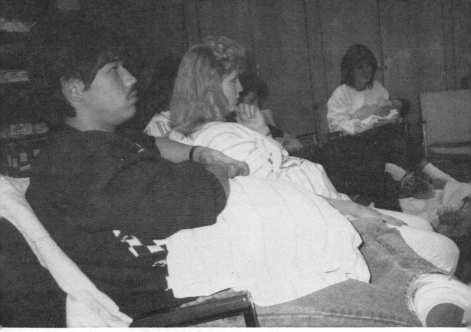

Pregnancy group, Fairbanks Counseling and Adoption

a pregnancy prevention program for school-age teens, community outreach, referrals, and home visits.

With initial funding from the Catholic Church, FCA is now affiliated with the local United Way. The pregnancy staff of four handles the program which also includes helping the teens complete their education, develop nurturing parenting skills, receive vocational training to become financially self-sufficient, and learn to communicate effectively with their families and community.

Bilingual Staff Provides Health Services

Holy Family Services, Weslaco, Texas, is located near the Texas-Mexico border, and provides health services to a large Hispanic population. During the first year, the bilingual staff served nearly one hundred pregnant teens, approximately twenty percent of the total patients served.

Classes for pregnant adolescents are conducted in a separate, well-equipped classroom. Curriculum is the Joseph P. Kennedy, Jr., Foundation's Community of Caring.

One of the most exciting aspects of the program is the newly constructed birthing center which offers women of the area an alternative to the traditional hospital delivery. The program is less expensive, and fees are on a sliding scale based on ability to pay.

Especially unique is the bartering system whereby low income families can arrange to reduce their amount of payment if family members work twenty hours painting, gardening, or helping with other chores.

The birthing center has duplex suites with four beds and a kitchenette. Family members are invited to accompany the young mothers, and to participate in the delivery if the patient chooses. At delivery time, medical back-up is provided through local physicians and hospitals.

Holy Family Services networks with schools, social agencies, and other health care providers. A hot line, called the "Care Line," has been added to deal with questions on teen pregnancy and sexuality.

Providing Residential Care

Maternity homes historically have provided residential and other services for single pregnant women. Today, many teen-agers continue to live at home throughout pregnancy, but residential programs are still needed for some teens.

A good maternity home generally provides opportunities for residents to develop essential life skills as well as shelter for pregnant teens who have limited options for housing at a difficult time in their lives.

Community Maternity Services, Albany, New York, provides a wide variety of adolescent pregnancy care and prevention services, including a maternity residence, a family development center for adolescent parents and their infants, an Infant Health Assessment Program, a Family Life Education Program, and an adoption and foster care program. A recent addition to CMS services is a program for boarder babies which provides a hospice for infants who have been abandoned in hospitals, many by young mothers who were drug abusers or the victims of AIDS.

Sr. Maureen Joyce, CMS Director, talked about the early development of the CMS maternity home in Albany:

*We started as the traditional maternity home in 1971.
New York had liberalized its abortion law, and people
figured maternity homes wouldn't be needed. If the pregnancy was a problem, abortion would take care of it, so
other homes in the state were closing.*

*At that time maternity homes were mostly for people
wanting anonymity, and almost all the residents were
considering adoption. They more or less stopped living as
far as continuing school or socializing were concerned.
They went away, had the baby, went home and said they'd
been taking care of a sick relative.*

*We knew in 1971 that wasn't appropriate, so we
decided we needed a much different kind of residential
care. It wasn't to be a hideout. It was to address our
clients' needs psychologically, academically, and
developmentally.*

*One of the basic things was that we certainly did not
specify residents needed to be considering adoption if they
stayed here. Adoption was fine, but it was not the criteria.*

*We decided it would be better for the young women in
our program if they could utilize community services
rather than having everything under our own roof as
maternity services had done previously. So we linked up
with resources in the community.*

*The young mothers attended either a traditional high
school, an alternative school, or a job-training center. We
helped each one develop an individual educational plan
using community resources. We also had a whole cadre of
tutors who came in to supplement, but not replace the
school program.*

*We did the same thing with health care. We wanted this
pregnancy to provide a model for her future pregnancies.
We wanted her to know how to go about getting a doctor
rather than receiving health care from people coming into
her home as had been done in maternity homes. So we
utilized physicians in the community. These young girls
make their own appointments and go to the doctor's
office, a normal way to get health care.*

*I think the most important part of residential care is
capitalizing on the fact that it is a group. We need to be
like a family, go over what happened during the day, be
involved in the conversation. It's the whole group process
— watching television, seeing something that needs to be
responded to. If you have a staff able to provide this kind
of support, they can see these young women through some
difficult times.*

Program for Homeless Pregnant Teens

Some pregnant teenagers have no home at all. **Capable
Adolescent Mothers (CAM)** of Crossroads Programs, Inc.,
Lumberton, New Jersey, is for these young people. Funded by
the Robert Wood Johnson Foundation, CAM is a residence for
homeless pregnant teens aged sixteen to eighteen. Teens may
come to CAM at any point in pregnancy and remain throughout
the child's first year.

The Department of Nursing at Temple University provides
staff training on pregnancy, labor and delivery, maternal/child
bonding, nutrition, and child growth and development. One
technique used by the staff is the videotaping of the mother/
infant feeding time. The instructor then plays the tape back with
the young mother which helps her recognize her baby's
feeding clues.

Community support has ranged from women's groups
knitting layettes to visiting nurses doing follow-up appraisals on
the babies' development, according to Dolores G. Martell,
Executive Director.

Staff works closely with child protective services, the health
community, the school system, welfare, potential employers,
and local churches and synagogues.

Intervention Makes a Difference

Pregnant teens are more likely to have health problems than
are older pregnant women. A high percentage of babies deliv-
ered to teenage mothers will be born too small and too soon.
About five percent of these tiny babies will have developmental
handicaps.

Research shows, however, that for teens sixteen and older, pregnancy need not be high-risk from a physical standpoint. Pregnant teens who do not smoke, do not consume alcohol or take drugs, who eat nutritious foods throughout pregnancy, and who receive good health care starting early in the pregnancy tend to have no more physical problems for themselves or their babies than do older women.

The problem, of course, is that without intervention which provides comprehensive services, many pregnant teens receive no health care until late in their pregnancies. Some receive none at all. Eating the foods needed for a healthy pregnancy requires a significant lifestyle change for many teens. So does abstaining from alcohol, drugs, and smoking.

High-quality intervention services greatly improve prenatal care and the health of mother and baby. Whether these services are coordinated through a school, health service, or social service agency, the importance lies in the accessibility and the comprehensiveness of the services provided to meet the unique needs of pregnant teenagers, services provided by caring, non-judgmental, and capable providers.

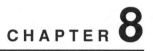

Helping
Teen Parents

The adolescent pregnancy prevention continuum includes helping young parents avoid some of the negative outcomes characteristically associated with too-early parenthood. In order to complete their education and job training, become good parents, and lead satisfying and productive lives, school-age parents usually need extra help.

Staying in school may appear impossible. Maintaining optimal health for themselves and their children may require special services. Even with family support (lacking for many teen parents), help in the form of comprehensive community services is needed.

Implementing school programs for school-age parents may be extremely difficult. Lack of child care and/or transportation may keep young parents from continuing their education. Cost, especially if child care is provided, may appear prohibitive. The community may not feel its adolescent parents "deserve" special services.

Thorough documentation of the need and informed, articulate community coalitions are essential. A creative and intense search for funding may be needed.

Health and social service personnel in your community may also feel overwhelmed dealing with the tremendous needs of teenage parents. Or they may be convinced that teenage parents need no special services because they feel programs designed for adults should be quite adequate.

Criteria for Care Programs

Because of the temporary nature of funding, programs and their comprehensiveness tend to expand or cut back in accordian-like fashion in relation to the current financial support. It is important that individuals designing adolescent pregnancy prevention and care programs think through the key elements necessary for a program's success at the beginning of the program planning process.

Success rarely just happens—it takes the right mix of thought, resourcefulness, committed people, and good planning and management.

Some key features for programs which have proved successful in serving teen parents were identified by Denise Polit in her book, *Building Self-Sufficiency: A Guide to Vocational and Employment Services for Teenage Parents* (1986: Humanalysis, Inc.). Polit included many of the following:

- **Comprehensiveness** means a complex array of educational, vocational, social, and health services are needed. These should be designed to meet the multiple needs of young men and women who are inexperienced in pursuing available community resources.
- **Support Services** include on-site child care, as well as some provision for transportation, counseling, meals, advocacy, and other identified needs.
- **Program Atmosphere,** to be inviting, means staff must work as a team, be sympathetic and supportive of the teens, and treat the teens with respect. Staff continually should focus on the enhancement of self-esteem for the young people in the program.

- **Peer Group Support** helps the teens develop a bond, a sense of belonging, and an identity with the program. It provides a forum for mutual problem-solving, and sets the norm for attendance and achievement.
- **Individualization** means the program providers know the teens, and the teens are involved in planning the program. Individualization maximizes opportunities for individual progress on a one-on-one basis, and provides for the diverse range of abilities in the teen participants. In short, it personalizes the program.
- **Program Schedule** needs flexibility as pregnant and parenting teens' lives often follow an irregular schedule. Consider whether open enrollment or fixed enrollment is preferable for the program's operation and for the participants.
- **Follow-up Services** are needed by many young parents after active program participation ceases. What type of on-going help, such as reunions or newsletters, will be provided? How can participants retain the feeling that they are cared about and are still a part of the program's "family"?
- **Staffing** emphasis must be on sensitive, caring, non-judgmental employed and/or volunteer staff who *enjoy* working with teens. Needed are individuals who can build rapport with the teens based upon mutual trust and respect. Many programs use mentors as role models and adult friends for the teens. Employed and volunteer staff need to be well trained in working with adolescents.
- **Involve teen clients** in a variety of ways. You'll be more successful if you "do with" rather than "do to" teens.
- **Holistic Approach** is vital because teens don't live in a vacuum. Programs should, whenever possible, involve the teen's partner and extended family to ensure that the needs of the total family unit are being addressed.
- **Case Management** is a component of many successful care programs. Generally, at least one staff member helps each participant meet her/his comprehensive needs. (The Teen Age Parent Program (TAPP) in San Francisco calls this individual a Continuous Counselor.)

- **Funding Diversification** is wise. Ideally, a program's funding should include a mix of public and private sources. Tapping multiple sources is time consuming and difficult, but provides greater assurance the program will continue even if one of the sources is not available in the future. Programs are expensive to operate. Funding must be carefully planned from the beginning.
- **Evaluation** should be an integral part of the program. Every program needs a process to collect and review appropriate information that will indicate if the program is achieving goals. Evaluation must be planned and implemented as a part of the program from the beginning.

Essential Core Services

In some programs, core services are offered on-site. Other programs provide these services through linkage agreements. Whichever plan of delivery is most feasible, the following services are needed by teen parents:
- Educational program for high school graduation including graduate equivalency program (GED preparation).
- Child care.
- Transportation.
- Vocational education/employment training.
- Consumer education/life management skills.
- Counseling including pregnancy alternatives.
- Parenting education.
- Health education including family planning.
- Prenatal education including childbirth education for pregnant clients.

In addition, English as a Second Language (ESL) classes, special education services, substance abuse prevention, and emergency intervention services should be provided.

Helping clients improve their self-esteem needs to pervade all services. Additional help may be needed in finding financial assistance, housing/shelter, and legal assistance in establishing paternity.

Ronda Simpson, **Teen Pregnancy/Teen Parent Coordinator Consultant, California Department of Education**, stressed

the need for the following special qualities in the staff working
with pregnant and parenting teens:

- Acceptance of self and others as sexual persons.
- Communicates effectively both verbally and non-verbally.
- Open-minded and non-judgmental with respect to values,
  attitudes, choices and behaviors which may differ from
  her/his own.
- Able to relate effectively to students with honesty, warmth
  and sensitivity.
- Has good listening skills.
- Can create a trusting supportive classroom atmosphere.
- Keeps communicated information confidential.
- Familiar with the physical aspects of pregnancy and
  understands the emotional and physical changes the
  student experiences.

Salem's Teen Parent Program

A number of social service agencies are providing creative
programs for pregnant and parenting teens, and some have
developed truly comprehensive offerings.

The **YWCA Teen Parent Program, Salem, Oregon,** serves
more than seven hundred pregnant and parenting teens, their
children, and their family members annually through a comprehensive, single-site program. The program coordinates support
services from numerous agencies in the community including
the Salem school district and the Marion County Department of
Public Health.

The Teen Parent Program, more than twenty years old,
provides education, child care, health care, counseling, employment, and young men's services on a year-round basis. Curriculum specialized to meet the needs of the teen parents includes a
mentor group and "Out on My Own," prenatal, child development, and parenting classes. Students and their children are
transported to and from the YWCA site by school district buses
equipped with infant seats and seat belts for the mothers. Breakfast and lunch are available on site for the parent and child.

Coordinated case management is inter-disciplinary and a key
feature in the success of the program. Recognizing that the

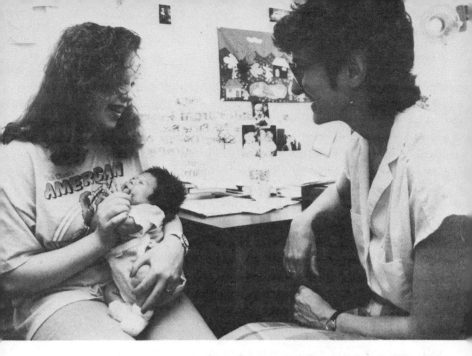

YWCA Teen Parent Program, Salem, Oregon

progress achieved over the course of the school year may be lost in a summer of isolation, the program has set up the "Mom and Tot Summer Program" which provides support groups, field trips, mom-tot swim classes, and respite care for infants. The latter gives the teen moms a few hours of free time each week.

Housed in the old Carnegie Library across the street from the State Capitol, the program encourages the young parents to participate in the legislative process by meeting with their representatives and watching the state legislature in action.

In recent years, students have purchased letter jackets that display "Teen Parents" on the back collar, and the names of the mother and child on the front. The young mothers are telling the community how much they appreciate the YWCA Teen Parent Program in a highly visible way, according to former director Sylvia Loftus.

Drop-in Center Offers Job Training

The Family Focus/Our Place Center, Evanston, Illinois, is a teen parent drop-in center featuring outreach, teen fathers, an Extended Family Project, one-on-one volunteer support through the "Partners Program," a junior high prevention project, on-site education and employment training, and child care.

Our Place has a reputation for constantly initiating new, creative adolescent pregnancy care and prevention activities such as the "Teen Cuisine" program, a food service employment training project for twenty-five low-income, single parents between the ages of fourteen and twenty-four years. Teen Cuisine provides work counseling, food service job skills training, and experiential employment to young male and female parents who are at high-risk of long-term unemployment and dependency upon public assistance.

"If you allow them to drop out, you're setting the pattern for failure."

Throughout the Teen Cuisine Project, parent trainees are provided with child care, academic tutoring, GED preparation, individual and group counseling, transportation stipends, referrals to other training/service programs, and other services available at the Our Place Center.

Delores Holmes, Director, explained:

When we opened Our Place ten years ago, we got static from the community, even from the school. I remember one counselor, a man, saying, "They had those babies. They need to stay home and take care of them." We told him, "Pay now or pay later. If you do this for these kids, they'll be able to make a living for themselves. If you allow them to drop out, you're setting the pattern for failure."

He's come a long way. He changed because he started looking at the kids as individuals.

If you encourage these young people a little, they go back to school and meet some of the goals he and we have for them, and more important, their goals. He didn't think they had any goals at all except to have babies. They demonstrated for him that they did want to do something with their lives.

*I think we've made such mistakes in dealing with poor
people in this country. There ought to be decent housing,
day care, educational services for all pregnant and
parenting teens, some way to keep them from dropping out
and being forced to survive on welfare. "Give them a fish
and they'll eat today. Teach them to fish and they can eat
forever."*

*Kids come here because they want to. For them the
attraction is our caring and our willingness to start where
the kids are. We say to young people, "We care about you,
and we want to work with you." That kind of statement
means that young people have to decide how to use us, or
whether to use us. They can walk in and walk right back
out. But nearly all the kids who drop in stay until they get
what they need, and then they keep coming back.*

Providing Case Management

Some health clinics realize that teens need special help, and
provide innovative services for young people.

An example of such a service for teen parents is **Connect,
A Program for Pregnant and Parenting Teens, Nampa,
Idaho.** Connect is a rural case management approach to services
for pregnant and parenting adolescents, and many core services
are provided within an existing rural primary care system. It is
based within Terry Reilly Health Services (TRHS), a private,
non-profit health care corporation in southwest Idaho.

Important to the work of Connect is its advisory committee,
according to Ann Sandven, Project Director. Among those on
this committee are a client and her mother, the superintendent of
schools, a local legislator, minister, vice principal in charge of
the teen parent school in Nampa, head of another alternative
school, a counselor from a small town high school, head of the
Health Department, Hispanic health educator, an obstetrical
nurse, two Terry Reilly Health Services Board members (one
is an elementary teacher and the other a retired elementary
principal), and someone from the business community.

"We need more business and media people, and they're hard
to get," Sandven commented. "We need more people who aren't

necessarily on our side in the beginning. By being on our advisory committee, they find out what we're doing, and that's important."

Sandven defines case management as continuous counseling, and says their system is a rural version of the one developed by TAPP in San Francisco. She explained:

> *Case management means the client has an advocate. She can get a temporary Medicaid card the day she walks in. She gets help in linking up with all the services she needs such as food stamps and WIC. She has a consistent person throughout as her case manager. She usually bonds with that person, and her case manager becomes a combination counselor, mom, advocate, friend, and visitor.*
>
> *A lot of the kids who aren't in Nampa are in the "outback," towns of five hundred to a thousand people, as well as in labor camps. They're pretty isolated. Many of them don't have phones, don't have friends, don't have cars, don't communicate with the rest of the world. The case manager is the person they can talk with, the person who is with them throughout pregnancy and the first two years of parenting.*
>
> *The case manager assesses her needs, makes out a game plan, and links her with the services she needs, then checks to see that she gets those services.*

Sandven said the not-in-school and not-in-health-care teens are the hardest to reach. As one approach, free pregnancy tests are done in the teen clinic one evening each week. Sandven feels this helps promote early prenatal care.

Group for Isolated Teen Mothers

Teresa Arana-Wood is an "Outback" case manager for Connect. She understands the isolation young parents feel who are home day after day, alone with their children. Most of her clients are not in school, they have no transportation, and they don't have telephones. Because they are not in school,

Arana-Wood helps them connect with a Graduate Equivalency Program (GED). She visits her clients every two weeks, and feels the isolation herself because she generally is in the Connect office only for weekly staff meetings and to get her files together early each morning.

Two years ago Arana-Wood decided to start a young mothers group. With the help of a volunteer co-facilitator, transportation and child care were organized. The two women transport most of their clients to the bi-weekly sessions in a church. Three volunteers from a pool of sixteen provide child care for the two-hour meetings. Arana-Wood explained:

I started the group out of desperation and with no extra funding. I was feeling burned out and overwhelmed with the amount of contact I felt these girls needed, and I didn't think I could do it all. They were missing a lot by not hearing other girls say, "I went through that . . ." They needed another young mom to talk with about a crying baby or an infant who spits up a lot.

I was also concerned about child abuse, alcohol, and other problems.

I tell them about community resources, and I bring in speakers. A lot of my time goes into planning and research.

We start the year with something informal and fun such as hair and makeup. Then we work into the threatening topics—sexual abuse, alcoholism, drug dependence, vocational training, and career counseling.

Each year new girls join us, so I wait until they feel part of it before we do a threatening session. We may do two sessions on these issues, then something fun like a field trip. I try to balance it so the group doesn't get burned out.

Some young women who graduated from the program at age nineteen wanted to stay, so I'm using them as peer counselors and role models. All of the girls are deeply involved in planning our sessions. They know this is their group, not mine.

Focusing on Native American Teen Parents

Teenage pregnancy and parenting is also the focus of **Tiospaye Teca (Young Families),** a program established in 1988 by **Rural America Initiatives** to address needs of young Native American families in **South and North Dakota.**

Tiospaye Teca was funded through Project Takoja II, a multi-site Teen Parent Program sponsored by Rural America through the Department of Health and Human Services. The South Dakota Department of Health, West River Community Health Center, is providing ongoing funding for the program. Tiospaye Teca is a comprehensive program serving more than fifty Native American teen families as well as additional non-Indians in its first year.

Rural America Initiatives has helped establish a number of community-based programs throughout the Dakotas, based on the organization's principle of local community empowerment, according to Anne Floden, Executive Director.

Teen parents receive assistance in accessing community services including referral to family planning services, pre- and postnatal care and classes, Women, Infant and Children Supplemental Nutrition (WIC), social services, Sioux San, and other agencies.

A community resource book has been compiled by Tiospaye Teca with more than 110 resources listed to help families with specific needs in Rapid City.

Parenting/Independent living classes are held for nine weeks in the summer. Jobs for teen parents have been provided through the Job Training Partnership Act (JTPA) Program. CHEERS, a four-day teen parent camp co-sponsored by Tiospaye Teca/Rural America Initiatives and West River Community Health Center, is held in the summer. Child care is provided on site.

MELD's Young Moms Offer Support

MELD's Young Moms (MYM), which originated in **Minnesota,** helps empower teen mothers through the period of transition from pregnancy into parenthood and self-sufficiency. Ann Ellwood founded MELD (known at that time as Minnesota Early Learning Design) in the early seventies. Designed first for groups of new parents generally, the group concept was soon refined to help teenage mothers as well.

An MYM group of ten to twenty teen moms meets weekly for two years. Mothers gather in groups according to their ages and the ages of their babies. Many are out of school and unemployed. At the MYM groups they learn they aren't alone, and they give and receive information, according to Ellwood.

Approximately fifty MYM groups are scattered across the United States. Each parent group facilitator plans the meetings and leads the group presentation with guidance from a project site coordinator.

Each MYM session begins with a meal which provides opportunity for informal teaching and role modeling. This allows time for the facilitators to note special individual and group needs—including the needs of the babies—in a relaxed atmosphere.

Curriculum for the weekly meetings covers health, nutrition, child development, child guidance, problem solving, education, and career development. Ellwood commented:

> *Facilitators are extremely important. We pair up two carefully selected volunteers, women who were themselves teenage mothers, women in their twenties who now have their lives in order and are still parents. It's not so hard to recruit. They're busy women, but they get a lot out of it themselves.*
>
> *Their training is extensive. It's done by the professional site coordinator who also calls the facilitator before each meeting, then again afterward to see how it went. The parent group facilitator knows she has someone to talk with immediately if she needs to.*

Sponsors for MYM groups, which house and support the program and site coordinator and assume most of the program's costs, may be a community agency, hospital, clinic, school, or government program. Co-sponsors such as benefactors, agencies, or churches, provide meeting space, food, transportation, or other donations.

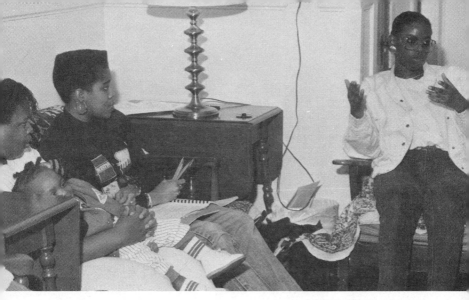

MELD's Young Moms

Combating Isolation with Home Visits

Another extremely rural area is poverty-stricken **St. Johnsbury, Vermont.** Operating since 1979, **Parent to Parent** program is an attempt to alleviate the social isolation and developmental disruptions that often accompany adolescent parenthood in this area. Northeast Kingdom Mental Health Services implemented Parent to Parent with training and technical assistance provided by the High Scope Education and Research Foundation, Ypsilanti, Michigan.

The home visitors, who volunteered their services during the early years of the program, are carefully selected, trained, and supervised, according to Winsome Hamilton, Director. Currently, each of six paraprofessionals visits six adolescent parents every week for at least a year. The home visitor and parent work as partners exchanging ideas and childrearing information, talking through problems, and discussing options. Some of the teen parents are in school, but the majority had dropped out before becoming pregnant.

The forty-hour staff training, according to Hamilton, focuses on three major areas:

> *We begin by discussing strategies for home visiting and the home visitor's role. I have them examine their own*

parenting attitudes and beliefs, and we talk a lot about mutual respect for the families we serve. One thing I stress is empowering these young women, not rescuing them. These young mothers are dynamic women. Although they may be currently rebelling or acting out against authority figures, they have tremendous potential. I impress upon the home visitors that we probably learn as much from the young parents as they learn from us.

Next we discuss available community services for the families, and how these systems work. And finally, we study child development so home visitors can plan appropriate activities to enhance parent/child interaction.

Vermont's Northeast Kingdom has a population of 56,000 scattered over 2,200 square miles, so outreach is important. Our home visitors put in incredible mileage, sometimes sixty miles for one visit. The visitors are scattered throughout the three-county area, and they work from their homes.

The home visit plans are designed to allow flexibility. The home visitor plans an activity for the child's developmental stage, but if she arrives and the teen mom is distraught by personal issues, the visitor is quickly able to adapt to the teen's needs that particular day. The home visitor plays the role of mentor, big sister, or surrogate parent as needed.

"Heart to Heart" for Abuse Victims

More than half the teenage mothers participating in a statewide survey sponsored by the Illinois Department of Children and Family Services said they had been sexually abused as children or forced into sex, some as early as age two. The average age for the first incidence of abuse was 11.5 years, and fifty percent of the 445 teenagers questioned reported that the same abuser had harassed them two to ten times. Similar findings are reported in research results from a Washington State study.

"Experiences were often coercive and sometimes aggressive, including rapes at knifepoint and boyfriends inviting their buddies to 'share' the frightened and confused victim," said Judith Musick, former Executive Director of the agency's Ounce of Prevention Fund.

The **Heart to Heart Program** was developed by the Illinois Ounce of Prevention Fund when young mothers in its **Parents Too Soon (PTS)** program began to disclose sexual abuse experiences as they talked together in their parent support groups. Plans for the program began when the Ounce of Prevention realized there was no existing model to help teen parents protect their children against sexual abuse, and that no model existed for protecting infants and toddlers from birth to age three.

Musick and Vicki Magee, Director of Parents Too Soon, sought to design a program which responded to the often hidden and secret nature of child sexual abuse. The name, "Heart to Heart," emphasized the close relationship needed between members of the group, as well as the need for a parent and child to speak openly.

Members of the Heart to Heart group feel comfortable with each other because they meet in an ongoing parent support group. Of the three facilitators, two are the regular parent support leaders. The other leader is a former child sexual abuse victim who cares deeply about helping adolescent mothers prevent child sexual abuse.

During the ten Heart to Heart meetings, the young women learn about three Illinois laws which protect children and provide legal remedies against violence. Participants also get information on social service resources they can use, and learn practical tips on keeping their children safe. Most importantly, by reconciling their own childhood experiences, they increase the likelihood that their relationships with their children will improve and that their children will be safe.

Housing for Young Mothers

Housing is a serious problem for many adolescent parents, and a few places offer group living for young mothers and their children. **The Vivian E. Washington Group Home, Baltimore, Maryland,** provides a home for up to eighteen mothers and their children. The goal of the program is to improve parenting, decision-making, and self-sufficiency skills through a family-oriented approach and setting. The teen mom must be in school, working, or in a job training program, and child care is provided. Similar to a dormitory setting, each parent must budget and manage her own money, do her own grocery shopping, and prepare breakfast and dinner for herself and her baby.

With the assistance of the local chapter of Delta Sigma Theta, the program was started by Vivian Washington, then director of the teen parent program for the Baltimore public schools. From the beginning, the program developed lots of community support from churches, civic and social groups, and other community organizations.

To create the family feeling, the program involves the parents of the teen moms, the fathers of the children, and other important people in the lives of the teens in many of the activities at the home. The program places a strong emphasis on the involvement of the baby's father by setting special visiting hours for fathers only.

Supporting Each Other

Teen mothers often report their friends vanish when they're pregnant or after delivery. Even if friends stand by them, the young mothers find they often can't go out as before because of lack of child care. Or they find they no longer have the same interests as those of their former friends.

The support of a group of other young mothers may bring a significant reduction in the isolation, boredom, and desperation sometimes experienced by young parents. The programs in this chapter illustrate a wide variety of approaches taken by communities across the country.

Each one is different from all the others, but each is alike in having a caring, empathetic staff determined to help prevent some of the problems associated with adolescent parenting. Over and over the young people report, "They made a difference in my life."

CHAPTER **9**

Providing
School Services

Research on school-age mothers' educational patterns indicates they are more likely to complete high school and delay subsequent pregnancies if they're enrolled in school during pregnancy and after birth. We must do all we can to help pregnant and parenting teens remain in school or, for those who have already dropped out, to return to school.

If your school district offers no special services to school-age parents, it may be because they honestly don't think they have teen parents in the district. Or they may be stereotyping young parents into a group of non-achieving, uninterested dropouts who wouldn't come to school anyhow. They may even have the old idea that "those girls" shouldn't be in school, either because they'll contaminate other students, or because they "made their bed and should lie in it!"

On the other hand, the administrators in your school district may simply be overwhelmed by the enormity of the task of attempting to help all young people stay in school. They may be convinced that they don't have the resources to provide special services.

Comprehensive school services, especially if on-site child care is provided, are expensive. Far more expensive, however, is permitting young parents to stay out of school with no job skills and little future except welfare dependency and more children. Programs which enable young families to be self-supporting are not expensive in the long run. Convincing your power structure of this seemingly obvious fact may not be easy, however, especially in this time of limited resources.

School-age parents need a variety of options. Some need child care in order to stay in their comprehensive high schools. Others have already dropped out of their home schools when they conceive or they do so during pregnancy or after childbirth. An alternative school setting may meet their needs. For some, home tutoring may be required.

An excellent resource which focuses on this issue is *A Stitch in Time: Helping Young Mothers Complete High School* by Elizabeth A. McGee with Susan Blank (1989: Academy for Educational Development).

Meeting Young Parents' Needs

Comprehensive services designed to meet young people's medical, social, and educational needs are optimal for pregnancy prevention and care services. For teens who already have children, comprehensive services are especially important for both the teen parent and her/his child. A scattering of school districts across the country provide comprehensive services for school-age parents at a single site, including on-site child care, a health clinic, counseling, job training, and transportation.

"Comprehensiveness, the staff, and community support are the most important factors in a school such as ours," commented Caroline Gaston, Principal, **New Futures School, Albuquerque, New Mexico.** She explained:

> *Many of our students don't enroll just because of the education. Some enroll because we say, "If you're preg-nant, come here to learn about your baby." Some come*

*for the health services, some for the counseling, some for
the social support, and some for the education.*

*Some of our students weren't able to learn in the
school of two thousand kids, and that was one of the
factors that led to their pregnancies. We need to have
different approaches to education for the at-risk child.
This may mean a lot more individualization of instruction,
perhaps using the discovery approach instead of lecturing.
Perhaps half of our teens need that kind of educational
approach.*

*The one-to-one relationship between the caring adult
and the student makes the difference. Too many alternative schools get the left-over teachers. Our students must
have the caring, understanding, and respectful relationship, the "I value you as an individual. You're going to be
a good parent."*

Case Management Strategy

Case management techniques are used to track, follow, and
counsel teen mothers and their families in the **Teen Age Preg-
nancy and Parenting Project (TAPP), San Francisco, Cali-
fornia**. The program is managed jointly by the Family Service
Agency of San Francisco and the San Francisco Unified School
District. Funding includes Federal Title XX Public Health
Funds, State Maternal Child Health Block Grant, United Way,
San Francisco Foundation, and the Ford Foundation.

TAPP serves pregnant and parenting women aged twelve to
eighteen. Clients don't have to attend school to receive TAPP
services, but helping young parents remain in or return to school
is a primary goal.

Each mother has a case plan requiring that she receive a
variety of health, education, and social services. These include
pregnancy testing, primary and preventive health services,
nutrition information, counseling, education, referrals to pediatric, mental health, family planning, STD screening, social
services, maternity homes, and child care. Young fathers are
also served by TAPP.

Amy Loomis, Director, explained the reasons behind TAPP:

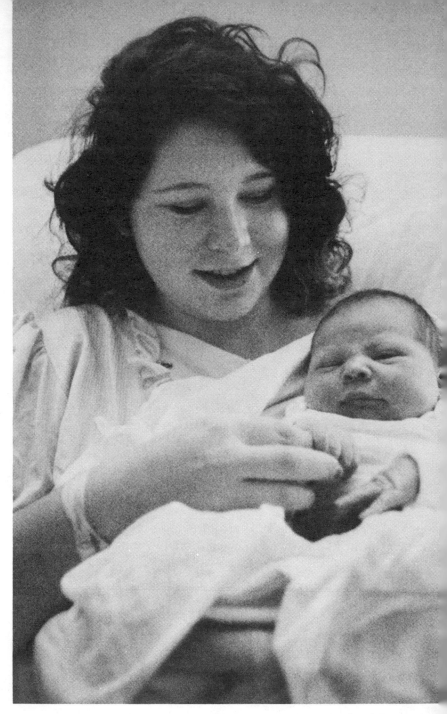

Photo by David Crawford

> *We had the Special Service Centers in San Francisco*
> *for pregnant teens, and they were great, but the young*
> *mothers could remain in the program only a semester*
> *after delivery. After that, the overwhelming majority*
> *simply dropped out of school. Without special help, they*
> *couldn't cope. They had no child care, no support, they*
> *didn't finish school, isolation set in, and repeat pregnancy*
> *often resulted.*
>
> *We needed comprehensive services for the parents, and*
> *in San Francisco, there was no way we could answer all*
> *these needs at a single site. So we developed the continu-*
> *ous counselor system. Rather than simple case manage-*
> *ment, it's a personal relationship over time, and that*
> *makes the difference.*

Several evaluations of TAPP have demonstrated that continuous case management improves staying in school and reduces
repeat birth rates significantly, according to Loomis.

Providing Comprehensive Services

The **Family Learning Center (FLC)** of **Leslie, Michigan**,
helps teen parents in the seven rural school districts of Ingham
County overcome their isolation by providing transportation to
the program, licensed child care, academic studies, programs for
vocational testing and placement, information on food and
clothing banks, counseling services, and community interagency
assistance.

Parenting skills are taught to both mothers and fathers, and
pregnant teens receive prenatal care.

The Center coordinates on-site and home visits by mental
health counselors and public health nurses. Fathers and extended
family members are included in counseling to build a supportive
environment for the teen parents.

Michigan State University places student teachers, student
nurses, and community service interns at the FLC for their
senior and postgraduate internships. A recent grant from the
Ford Foundation allowed the FLC to expand its facilities. The
grant also provided matching support for a scholarship fund for

outstanding Center graduates who wish to pursue vocational training or academic studies at community colleges and universities in the area.

Jean Ekins, Director of the Family Learning Center, says, "The results of the program have evolved into more than any of us had initially dreamed when we started the program in 1975. The percentage of our seniors who graduate is well over ninety percent per school year. With small classes and teacher attention, the grade points of our students remain consistently higher than when they were in traditional school, and the families we have touched throughout the years are now providing a large base of support."

Retrieving Dropouts Through Outreach

Many pregnant teenagers are not enrolled in school. Some drop out before they become pregnant while others quit attending school after they realize they've conceived. School programs which serve only those students already enrolled in school miss many potential clients.

Getting dropouts back into the education system is an important goal for **Adolescent Family Education, Tucson, Arizona,** according to Sherry Betts, Director. This is a change in focus from 1965 when the program was started strictly as an academic center. Currently, an average of 140 students are enrolled at one time in this alternative school, with a total of about 250 per year.

The regular senior and junior high courses plus electives are offered as well as special classes in parenting and prenatal health. The program has a strong career and work experience component. A mentor program is also provided for students.

A dozen years ago when Betts joined the program, most of the students were Anglo and a few were African American. Betts recalled there were no Native Americans and only a sprinkling of Hispanic students at that time:

Almost all the Hispanic and Native American girls who became pregnant dropped out of school, partly because of embarrassment, but we also discovered the district made it difficult for kids to continue school during pregnancy.

"Today sixty percent of our population are retrieved dropouts."

We did a couple of things. We developed a strong network in the community. We knew that when they dropped out, they didn't say, "I'm pregnant." They simply disappeared. So our nurse did intensive outreach to all prenatal health providers, and we identified the "lost" students. The nurse visited them at home, and we invited the dropouts and their parents in to see our program and to talk with us. Gradually we were able to increase our minority enrollment. Now a majority of our students are Hispanic.

By working through social service agencies where low-income kids would go, we began to draw a lot of young people who were not enrolled in school. Before this, many of the students in the program came directly from the other schools. Today, sixty percent of our population are retrieved dropouts.

As this happened, the needs of our students changed. We weren't dealing only with the normal hassles of families accepting the pregnancy, getting medical care, and making plans for the baby. We began to have more and more kids with more complex problems. Some were homeless, and some had been in the criminal justice system, kids who fit the description of the chronic dropout who happens to be pregnant.

To meet these needs, we had to expand our services. That's how we got into the career component of our program, and that's why we began to offer breakfast as well as lunch—we had kids who came to school in order to eat.

If a community is going to start a program, they need to decide on their target population. Their population will be very different if they simply work with a group of young people in school who happen to get pregnant than if they try to service all of the young people in the community

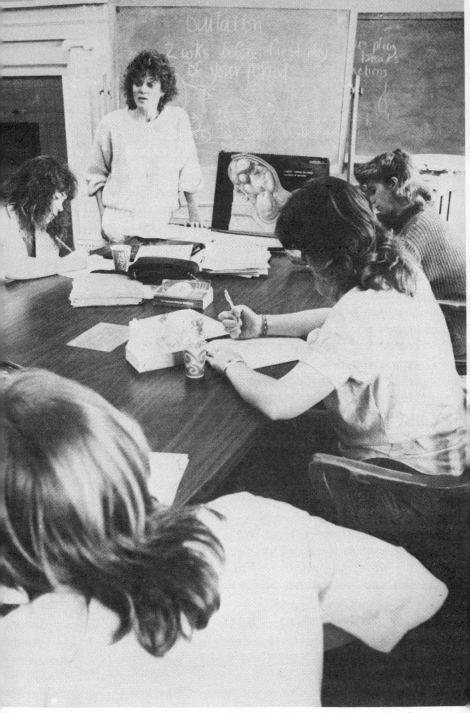

YWCA Teen Parent Program, Salem, Oregon

*who are getting pregnant and having babies. It's a broad
population and may mean you can't have the program
only on a high school campus.*

*If they dropped out of school because of their prob-
lems, they aren't going back to that campus to get their
needs met.*

Sometimes districts decide to mainstream pregnant and
parenting students because of the stigma associated with self-
contained programs, or, as may happen more often, because
mainstreaming may be less expensive. Pregnant and parenting
teens include a wide variety of young people, however, and
offering both mainstreaming and special programs is probably
the best approach.

Communities-in-Schools Approach

The **St. John's Teenage Parent Program, Austin, Texas,** is
a self-contained school serving pregnant teens and young
mothers for three months after delivery. Eight certified secondary teachers serve an enrollment varying from 85 to 110. Child
care is available there and on two other high school campuses in
the city, according to Tina Juarez, Director.

Juarez commented on the need for special services in the
schools:

*About a quarter of our students had already dropped
out of school when they came here. I feel some of these
kids really need a separate program. Not everybody feels
comfortable with being pregnant, especially toward the
end when they get so big and clumsy. Here everyone is in
the same situation.*

*If she's behind grade level, and about eighty-five
percent of our students are, our smaller classes give her a
chance to improve her grades and perhaps move ahead
faster than she might on the regular campus. When she
leaves here, we help her enroll in the regular school, an
alternative school, or in job skills classes or, if necessary,
home study.*

Communities in Schools (CIS), Austin, Texas, targeted the teen parent population as a group needing case management, focusing on teen parents in comprehensive schools and school-age dropouts as well as students in the St. John's Teenage Parent Program.

"When the CIS counselor is here, we do a lot of job training and career planning. A person from the Texas Employment State Commission works with us, and she pounds the streets trying to find employers who might hire our students during the summer," Juarez reported.

Melanie Lockhart, now Executive Director of the Texas Association Concerned with School-Age Parenthood (TACSAP), headed the CIS program in Austin for two years. She described the services:

> *We started with Job Training Partnership Act (JTPA) and County Human Resources money. We went to the Teenage Parent Alternative School and said we'd work with the girls, and we'd follow them when they went back to the regular school. I used a staff of interns from the University of Texas, Austin, School of Social Work. Our Communities in Schools model is to have a skeleton staff supplemented with university interns and community people.*
>
> *Basically, we provided case managers for the teen parents. We included husbands and boyfriends whenever possible—they were always welcome at support groups and in counseling.*
>
> *We continued working with those who dropped out of school. We spent a great deal of time on home visits. It was important to contact them at school, but we felt strongly about getting to know the members of their families. My interns saw the kids at least once a week, often at home.*
>
> *I think a strong case management system makes a big difference. We provided several levels of service, from the client who simply needed a mentor and a buddy to those kids who needed a lot more help.*

School Program Emphasizes Job Training

Building self-sufficiency skills through employment training and placement programs has become an increasingly important program piece in serving pregnant and parenting teens. Barbara Cambridge, past president of the Texas Association Concerned with School-Age Parents (TACSAP) and vice chair of the Impact '88 Youth-at-Risk committee in Dallas, says, "There have been a wide variety of job-related programs for young people in recent years. But to have a lasting impact, we need to make sure young people receive meaningful training for meaningful jobs."

The Boulder Valley Schools **Teen Parenting Program, Boulder, Colorado**, started as a self-contained program located at an elementary school. In 1987 it was moved to Fairview High School in order more fully to integrate students into the traditional secondary school environment. A major reason for the move was to provide more opportunities for teen parents to participate in vocational education and to find jobs. In addition to being assisted with career exploration and job skills, teen parents are encouraged to enroll in job training programs at the Boulder Area Vocational Technical Center.

This partnership project retrieved thirty dropouts in its first few months of operation.

Boulder County Private Industry Partnership (BCPIP) works closely with the teen parents, and provides job preparation training followed by job placement. About half the students participate in BCPIP's summer program which includes summer school and full or part-time employment.

A dropout retrieval coordinator was hired in 1988 under a grant from the Governor's Job Training office to get teen parents back in school, to give them job development and training assistance, and to re-enroll them in general and/or vocational training programs. This partnership project of the Boulder Valley School District, St. Vrain School District, and BCPIP had retrieved thirty dropouts in its first few months of operation. To achieve this success, twenty-four contacts were made with county agencies such as the Boulder County Health Department, Peoples Clinic, San Juan Health Clinic, WIC, YMCA Teen Center, and Emergency Family Assistance. At each agency, a contact person was established who was given referral forms and brochures along with the request to refer teen parents to the Teen Parenting Program.

Gloria Parmerlee-Greiner, Teen Parenting Program Director, credits the program's success to its active advisory board. Individuals from child care and health care, and from business and industry are involved. "That's your PR for the community," she commented.

GRADS Provides Help

Ohio offers the **GRADS (Graduation, Reality, and Dual-Role Skills)** program in many school districts throughout the state. This is an in-school, secondary program for pregnant and parenting students which is funded through the state Vocational Education/Home Economics office. Follow-up studies show good results, according to Gene Todd, GRADS state supervisor. The retention rate has ranged from eighty-four to ninety percent since the program began in 1980.

A GRADS program is organized in either of two ways: It may be a program in which one GRADS teacher-coordinator teaches GRADS classes at one or two high schools, or the GRADS teacher-coordinator may teach the classes at an Area Vocational School site as well as at local feeder schools. During the 1988-89 school year, 119 GRADS teachers taught in 211 school districts at 287 schools with more than five thousand students enrolled.

In addition to teaching classes, teachers are allowed time to meet with providers of community services, make home and hospital visits, conference with students, and work with school personnel.

The average number of contacts made by one teacher within the last school year included seventy-three home/hospital visits, 236 GRADS conferences, 225 teacher/guidance contacts, ninety-three administrative contacts, ninety parent contacts, 124 non-GRAD student conferences, 137 agency contacts, and thirteen speaking engagements. The average number of students per teacher per year is fifty-one.

"You can't have the program with the schools only. You have to have the total community connection," Todd stressed.

Single Parent and Homemaker Grants helped provide child care and transportation for GRADS students. Day care moneys are provided for at-school day care, community contract day care, or in-home day care. Transportation moneys are used for travel of parent and child from home to day care, parent to school and return to day care, and parent and child to their home.

"Research shows that these young people must gain control of their lives, and they have to do it themselves with support from their teachers, school, family and community. They have to learn to solve their own problems successfully, and when that happens, their self-esteem goes up and they move ahead. That's the real crux of the issue," Todd pointed out.

Home Economics Offers Special Class

Not only in Ohio, but across the country Home Economics teachers are taking the lead in providing special services for pregnant and parenting students in their home schools. The **Teen Parent Progam** at **Marshalltown High School, Marshalltown, Iowa,** is an example.

*"The students said if it weren't
for the special services,
they wouldn't be in school."*

This small and comprehensive program is funded by the local district with support services provided by the Iowa Department of Education with funds from the Carl Perkins Act. According to Joyce Keller Huff, Coordinator, the program started with two homebound tutors in the seventies. The students and teacher started meeting in the afternoon at school, and from there it evolved into students attending regular classes at the high school plus a special class, Positive Parenting, taught by Huff. Focus is vocational, and several fathers have enrolled in the class.

Volunteers are an important part of the program. The high school provides volunteer tutors as needed, and the YWCA operates a weekly support group. Another volunteer group helps the young women through labor and delivery. Several local service clubs and churches have also provided help with clothing, housing, child care needs, baby equipment, Christmas gifts, and food items.

The district has provided released time for Huff to write curriculum for the program. Fifty percent of her teaching time is scheduled for the Teen Parent Program which allows time for coordinating the many community services and child care, visits to her students' homes, and other support.

"One year the district considered cutting the program," she recalled. "We talked with the students, and they said if it weren't for the special services, they wouldn't be in school. This meant we were keeping about twelve students on the roll who wouldn't otherwise be in school.

"The district figured that reimburses the half-time teaching position. It's got to be dollars and cents."

Native American Teen Parent Program

A special self-contained program for pregnant and parenting students is offered through the **Young Mothers Program, Blackfeet Reservation, Browning, Montana**. As in some other school districts, the program grew out of a concern for homebound pregnant students.

Located across the street from the high school, students may enter the YMP two months before delivery, and remain for two months after their babies are born.

Janet Guardipee, teacher, coordinates community speakers, provides tutoring for the students, and visits them in their homes. Babies three weeks to two years of age are cared for in the nursery, and the young mothers attend a parenting class. They also work in the nursery each day in addition to their academic classes at the high school.

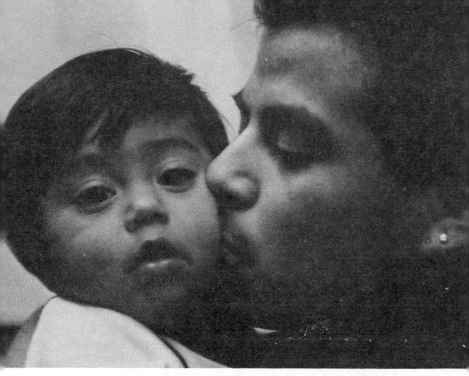

Photo by David Crawford

The fathers are welcome to be with their babies before school, at lunch time, and after school, according to Guardipee. A father's group is coordinated by a counselor and a teacher at the high school.

Camper Is Site for Independent Study

Ideally, school-age parents will have access to comprehensive services in a group setting with their peers. In many areas, however, these services aren't available.

In addition, teen parents vary as much as the rest of the school-age population, and some may prefer to study independently at home. Or she may be home because her school provides no transportation for herself and her child, and she has no way to get there.

The **Santa Clara, California, County Office of Education** has an unusual and workable plan for at-home parents—a twenty-foot motor home driven by **Independent Study** teacher Lois Joesten. Joesten takes the school vehicle to her students. She parks at the curb, and for an hour she and her student work at a small dinette table surrounded by textbooks, file boxes, and packets of study materials.

"I encourage them to call me at home.
We can work out the math on the phone."

If there is no one else to watch the baby when Joesten arrives, the mother brings him/her into the motor home to play with the wicker basket full of balls, rattles, and pull toys. Joesten even stocks teething biscuits for fussy babies.

Under the Independent Study guidelines, each student is expected to complete a minimum of twenty hours of homework each week. Most students work on basic skills in addition to parenting assignments. Students who stick with the program can earn a regular high school diploma without ever stepping into a traditional classroom again. Joesten discussed the program:

> *It's no fun to sit twenty hours a week working on your own time with no one standing over you saying, "Work. Work." It takes a lot of self motivation, and I come around once a week to help her over the rough spots.*
>
> *I use a holistic approach with the girls. They need to be in touch with bonding with the baby, relationships with their families, community services, and, last but not least, the academics. I encourage them to call me at home. We can work out the math on the phone.*
>
> *If I show up at the appointed time, and my student is obviously upset and has had a bad week, we talk about that first. Listening without making judgment statements is key. These young women are emotionally fragile, and they need someone to listen and to care. After that's out of the way, we turn to the weekly academic assignments.*

Itinerant Worker for Three Counties

In some rural areas, school districts combine to offer services to pregnant and parenting teens. Itinerant social worker Helen Guisler operates the **Teen Pregnancy and Parenting Program, McVeytown, Pennsylvania.** Funded through the State

Department of Education, the local districts, and Tuscarora Intermediate Unit II, the program serves three rural counties including seven school districts.

Guisler drives 50-100 miles daily as she visits students at twelve schools. She explained her approach:

> *Schedules are arranged in two-week cycles. In one school I may have two students, in another, twenty-five. I spend two hours at some schools, two days in another. We meet with students individually, about 110 this year, and on a group basis in their schools and homes. We do a lot of career planning, decision-making about the future, discussions of continuing school, jobs, marriage.*
>
> *There is no special program in the home schools except us. Primarily we provide supportive counseling, health education, parenting education, and encourage students to stay in school and finish their education.*
>
> *We also do a lot of referrals to community agencies, and in several schools run a monthly support group where all the kids at one school get together. Once a year we have a day-long workshop for students from seven schools. We'd do that more often if transportation weren't such a problem.*
>
> *There is an annual evaluation of the program, and the thing students seem to appreciate most is having one person who is especially interested in and provides support to them.*

Comprehensiveness Is Crucial

Whether they live in a rural, urban or suburban community, teen parents need special services, and they need those services to be as comprehensive as possible. Val echos comments made by most of the young mothers we interviewed, comments expressing the great need these young mothers have for school services:

> *I'm so supportive of Young Families. It gave me a support system, and I knew other girls who were going*

through some of the same things I was. Also parenting skills—when you're fourteen, you don't know much about parenting. The program also helped my self-esteem. They teach you that you made a mistake, but you're still an okay person. If Young Families hadn't been there, I probably wouldn't have stayed in school.

I'll graduate in June and I'm planning to go on to college. I'll have Rozanne with me. She's wonderful—she can hit a baseball like you wouldn't believe.

Some programs, such as some alternative schools, offer health and social services on site along with educational and vocational courses. Others provide for comprehensiveness through an extensive case management approach, a system which may be coordinated through health services, social service agencies, or the school.

As you set goals for your efforts in helping young parents, remember you'll undoubtedly be more effective if you work toward providing comprehensive services. To overcome the possible disadvantages of becoming a parent too soon, young people need help in becoming physically, emotionally, and mentally healthy, educated adults.

The community that provides the comprehensive services needed to help young people realize their goals is the community most likely to win the battle against the negative consequences of too-early parenting.

CHAPTER 10

Caring
For the Next Generation

A truly comprehensive approach to reflect the adolescent pregnancy prevention continuum effectively in a local community includes services for the children of the teen parents. Attitudes related to self concept, security, feeling loved, a sense of belonging, and a sense of worth begin to be established from the earliest years. Values are formed during these years. Role models of adults after whom the child will pattern his/her life are mirrored in the child's play. An understanding of what it means to be male or female in the home, community, and society is developed.

Babies at Risk

One of every six children in the United States is born to a mother who is a teenager. Many of these young mothers are uneducated, unskilled, and unmarried. Their children are at-risk for prematurity, low birth weight, and birth defects. They are more likely to have physical, emotional and intellectual handi-caps than are children born to mothers in their twenties.

Even if the baby is healthy at birth, the low socioeconomic level in the homes of many school-age parents affects the achievement levels and the behavior of their offspring, some-times handicapping them before they enter school. Social disadvantages of the mother's environment are more likely to be the cause of these problems than are biological or genetic factors.

The children of teenage parents are more likely to have special needs than are children of older parents, but intervention can make a difference. With assistance, young mothers and fathers can learn to prevent further early childbearing. They can provide appropriate nurturing, nutrition, stimulation, and train-ing for their youngsters to keep them from suffering emotional, behavioral and educational damage.

The young parents can understand the importance of helping their children develop high self-esteem providing their own needs in this area are met.

Learning to Be a Parent

Becoming a parent can be an exciting *and* stressful experi-ence for people of all ages. Lack of sleep, increased expenses, losing control of one's personal schedule, spending waking hours meeting the demands of a tiny infant, and adjusting to a sudden, major change in life's priorities leave most parents physically and mentally exhausted for the first weeks and months following the birth of a baby.

For a teen parent, add to that list isolation from friends, lack of financial resources, lack of transportation, and academic demands that may not be related to the student parent's immedi-ate or future needs. These demands, particularly for a teen parent who is still working through the developmental stages of adolescence, create a stress level that's off the charts.

Good parenting is not instinctive. It is a learned skill—learned by modeling others, reading, talking, asking advice, and understanding the basic human needs for love, security, and a sense of belonging.

Good parenting involves understanding how to discipline in appropriate, positive ways. Good parenting involves understanding the child's developmental stages and his/her emotional, psychological, mental and physical needs at each stage. It involves developing the patience and the maturity to deal with the never-ending tasks of parenting.

Basic to being a good parent is one's own sense of self-worth. Too often teen parents are assumed to be poor parents, too immature to handle the role. The young mother's own parents may be convinced she can't parent their grandchild adequately, so they take much of the responsibility for doing so. Other adults in the young parent's life may disapprove of her parenting efforts. Her doctor or her social worker may criticize her parenting style, or they may simply assume she's not doing well. She, in turn, can feel their disapproval.

Sadly, this disapproval may prove to be a self-fulfilling prophecy. People around her think she's not a good parent—and she fulfills their expectations by not being a good parent.

The young father may feel even more criticism of his parenting efforts. As a result, he may simply retreat from his new family, and remain a father only in a biological sense.

Teaching Parenting to Teen Parents

To repeat, good parenting is not automatic. It is an art and a skill, something most of us must learn. Some teen parents have already practiced parenting through taking responsibility for younger siblings, but others have had little or no chance to work with babies and small children. Even if they haven't experienced diapering and bathing a baby, however, most young parents will learn these techniques easily. It's the day-in, day-out consistent and constant loving care required by a baby that may be difficult to provide.

Many older parents and perhaps most teenage parents can profit from involvement in a well-taught parenting class. Teaching parenting to school-age parents must be one of the most relevant assignments a teacher can have because most—probably all—young parents *want* to be good parents. Teen parents, fathers and mothers, need help in achieving that goal.

Ideally, fathers as well as mothers are involved in learning to become the good parents they want to be. While most of the programs described in this chapter work mainly with young mothers, any program dealing with parenting should plan to include the fathers whenever possible and appropriate.

Burton White, author and child development expert, suggests the most important time for learning in a person's life is the first three years after birth. If a child is parented well during this period, s/he is likely to become a coping, self-sufficient person. In other words, helping a teenage parent learn the art and skills of parenting while her/his child is an infant/toddler is likely to have a positive effect on the child for many years.

The teenage parent can learn best if she is respected as a caring loving parent. Sally McCullough, head teacher of the **Tracy High School Infant Center, Cerritos, California**, for many years, stresses that the expert on her own baby is the young mother herself. That assumption is the foundation of parenting education at Tracy. McCullough stated:

> *Even in the case of a fifteen-year-old, if she has a baby and has cared for that baby in a loving way, she knows a lot about that child even if she isn't able to verbalize the hows and whys of good parenting. For example, she knows how to hold her baby so he'll be most comfortable.*
>
> *The baby and the mother are a natural unit, and if we respect and build on that unit, the mother is more able to care for the baby. But if we come barging in from the outside and say, "I know all about this baby, and you must do it my way," we're defeating the mother, making her feel inadequate. We undermine the very thing we want to support.*
>
> *We can still instruct the mother even though we support this bonding—if she feels we're on her side.*

The Tracy Infant Center was started in 1974, two years after the Teen Mother Program at Tracy High School began operation. McCullough explained that the Infant Center was developed because too many students were remaining in school during pregnancy, only to drop out after childbirth because they had no one to care for the baby:

> *We knew we had to have child care on campus if we expected the young mothers to remain in school. We soon realized two other important reasons for having child care here.*
>
> *Not only could the young parent stay in school, but her child was getting a good start because of our developmental approach to day care. And in addition, through the modeling of the Infant Center staff and the parenting class held daily, the young mothers' parenting skills improved remarkably.*

McCullough maintains that the parenting abilities of young mothers involved in the Infant Center starting soon after the birth of their babies were noticeably greater than those of young mothers enrolling in the program a year or so after childbirth.

Breaking the Cycle

Responding to the teen parent's child is most important, Judy Peterson, Director, **BETA, Orlando, Florida,** believes:

> *We've got to keep this problem (too-early pregnancy) from rolling over onto the child, and I think we can do it. I don't want her child to drop out of school. I can live with one generation having problems, but it would break my heart to see them thrown over onto the child. That's what we're trying to help prevent.*

"Breaking the Cycle" is BETA's term for the comprehensive services provided there for pregnant and parenting teens. The school is operated by the Orange County Public School system for students in grades six to twelve. BETA, a private organization, offers a residence for young women and their children. BETA also provides child care and parenting classes. The counseling program encompasses both the public school and the BETA components.

The BETA nursery is a large sunny room with high peaked windows. Twenty-one cribs line one wall, each with a mirror at the wall end, clear plexiglass at the other. Babies spend little waking time in bed, but when they do, they see either themselves in the mirror or they can look out at the big room. At one end of the room is a circle of rocking chairs. At the other end is a big thick mat covered with heavy vinyl printed with red, blue and green designs.

"We designed the room so babies don't spend a lot of time in bed," Peterson commented. "Much of the time they're interacting with volunteers—making eye contact, body contact. We hold them close, we talk to them, we touch their cheeks."

Nursery staff includes professionals trained in child development and pediatric nursing, but most of the caregivers are volunteers, according to Peterson:

> *We try to have almost a one-to-one ratio with the babies. It's a teaching nursery. Stats tell us that babies of teen moms lag in communication and cognitive skills. We work intensively with our babies to keep them at developmental level.*
>
> *We use two instruments, the Denver Developmental Scale and the NCAST to assess what is happening with the babies and their mothers. These aren't to place blame or to make the mom feel guilty. Rather, they give us guidance for our work. NCAST is an assessment tool for mother/ child interaction. How is that mom responding to that baby? That's something we need to look at.*

The BETA child development course consists of mothers and babies working together, according to Peterson:

> *In the afternoons the mothers come into the nursery. They're on the mat with their babies, and we go through exercises and activities that reinforce the baby's growth to the next level.*
>
> *We videotape the mothers and babies as they interact with each other. Then, at the end of class, we play the tape. Staff doesn't comment, but the mothers are trained*

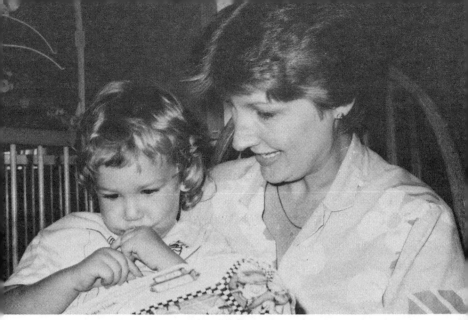

BETA's Breaking the Cycle, Orlando, Florida

to look for eye contact during feeding, and signs of disengagement on the baby's part indicating he's tired. Mothers learn the teachable moment for their children.

That's our child development course. It's a hands-on, low-key method. Nobody says, "You shouldn't be doing that." "You aren't doing a good job." "You failed the test." Instead, they're learning hands-on parenting with good modeling and lots of encouragement within a support group.

I'm convinced that ninety-nine percent of breaking the cycle is raising that mother's self-image. If she values herself, she values her child.

Education Lags Without Child Care

Each year nearly 500,000 teens give birth. Statistics reveal that sixty-one percent of the AFDC (Aid to Families with Dependent Children) grants go to families headed by a woman who first gave birth as a teenager. Need for welfare support is often linked with lack of education, and many teenage parents cannot continue their education because of lack of child care. Completing at least a high school education is an important factor in developing self-sufficiency.

John Winn, Education Policy Director, Office of Policy Research and Improvement, **Florida Department of Education,** recently did a survey in Florida which showed that lack of child care was the major barrier to young people completing their education. He commented:

> *Of course we knew that, but this provided the data. Without convenient child care close to the student's home school, she'll drop out, and most child care programs are at Teen Parent Program sites. These are students likely to be economically disadvantaged, and they have no child care available.*
>
> *As long as we have human beings, we'll have teenage pregnancy. We need support systems that don't reinforce negative behavior, but once a youth, through too-early pregnancy, has reduced her odds of being a productive citizen, we need to provide care programs to help her go on.*
>
> *If you provide good comprehensive programs, they enroll. If we had empty child care programs around the state, we could say they aren't interested. But that's not happening.*

According to Winn, there are three main reasons to provide child care for the children of teen parents:
1) To keep the school-age parent in school to complete his/her education.
2) To give the child of the teen parent a healthy start—emotionally, mentally, and physically.
3) To develop the teen parents' skills in good parenting.

Ann M. Wilson, Director of the **New Jersey Network on Adolescent Pregnancy,** is a member of the New Jersey Child Care Advisory Council. She, too, stressed the need for school-based child care:

> *Without child care, teen parents don't go back to school. Thirty-year-old mothers have trouble finding day care, then getting up at 6 a.m. to get themselves and their*

*babies to the care center, then themselves to work. For a
fifteen-year-old, it's impossible.*

*Our experience is that school-age parents need some-
thing different. They need help with child care, yes, but
they also need child care classes and support groups. It's
similar to teens being involved in family planning clinics.
They walk into a room full of thirty-year-olds, and they'll
turn right around and walk out.*

*The best possible scenario is school-based child care.
We know they have to get that diploma, and to make this
possible, they have to have child care.*

*I think the time has come for child care. Older parents
are demanding it, and the challenge is to bring the teen
parents along. If we don't help them finish school, we'll
get the bill later in welfare.*

Helpful Resources

*In School Together: School-based Child Care Serving Student
Mothers* by Michele Cahill, J. Lynne White, David Lowe, and
Lauren E. Jacobs (1987: Academy for Educational Development) is a handbook detailing the development of child care
programs. It's an extremely useful how-to book which provides
information on design, staff, program, funding, and other aspects
of providing child care services for school-age parents.

The Wellesley College Center for Research on Women
prepared a directory of child care programs serving teen parents
called *Learning Together: Child Care Programs for Teen
Parents* (1989: Wellesley College). The directory includes descriptions of more than three hundred programs across the
country, and provides a wealth of information regarding services
offered, funding sources, and contact persons.

Expense of Providing Child Care

Providing developmental care for infants is expensive.
Required staffing may be as high as one adult per three or four
babies. Yet this is the time child care is most needed by
young parents.

Infant centers generally seek multiple funding sources to maintain their programs. Possible sources include federal programs such as Job Training and Partnership Act (JTPA), state agencies, local school districts, local agencies and organizations, United Way, foundations, businesses, and personal donations.

Schools wishing to provide day care may be too crowded already. If space is available, funds are needed for renovation. Infant care requires a specialized facility with sinks in the room, fenced play yard adjacent to the child care room, fire doors, and other unique features. Temporary buildings are sometimes used on or near school grounds.

Most teen parents in the United States cannot pay full fees for infant care. Many can pay practically nothing, so most of the cost must be covered by other sources.

Most of the young mothers in the **Carlsbad, New Mexico, AWARE** program are income-eligible for child care at school at no cost. Charges for those not eligible for free child care are prorated based on their income.

However, Winn Van Cleave, AWARE Program Director, observed that those being charged fees could barely afford them, so they worked out a system which she and those in the program consider more fair.

"We tell them nobody pays, but everybody shares in the work. To raise funds, we have car washes and bake sales, and this money is used for the necessary student payments," she explained.

While this approach doesn't support the major financial needs of the child care center, it helps all the young parents understand something about the costs involved in providing child care.

Transportation may be a problem in child care planning. Sometimes school districts don't want the liability of transporting babies. Infant seats are needed in buses, and these are costly. Yet many places lack access to public transportation. Transportation may be especially difficult in rural areas.

In Carlsbad, transportation is a problem, according to Van Cleave. With the backing of her active Advisory Board, she wrote a letter to the editor of the local paper explaining their need for a fifteen-passenger van. A private foundation donated

$9,000, and $8,000 was provided by United Way. Small donations from the community totaled an additional $5,000. The van, equipped with eight infant seats, picks up students and babies at home as needed, and transports the young mothers between the AWARE site and their home schools.

Involving Seniors in Child Care Service

Foster grandparents from **ACTION** are employed in the child care center at **St. John's Teenage Parent Program (TAP), Austin, Texas.** ACTION is a federally funded program for women and men over the age of seventy.

"They're paid a small stipend, and we provide lunch for them. Transportation is by city bus," explained Tina Juarez, St. John's TAP director. "We do staff development with the foster grandparents. Usually each infant is assigned to a specific grandmother, and we encourage the baby's mother to go first to the grandmother with her questions.

"The students get along well with them. We've been utilizing foster grandparents for six years, and three of them have been with us all those years."

A child development center at the Orangeburg-Calhoun Technical College, **Orangeburg, South Carolina,** was opened in 1988 for children of teenage mothers on public assistance. **The Intergenerational Child Development Center,** staffed in part by senior citizens, is a pilot program to enable AFDC and income-eligible mothers to return to school or get a job with the ultimate goal of being self-supporting.

Designed to serve a maximum of fifty children from the ages of six weeks through five years, the Center is a joint project of the Governor's Office, Orangeburg-Calhoun Technical College, the State Health and Human Services Finance Commission, and the State Commission on the Aging.

The program is designed to meet the specific needs of each of the population groups it includes. The elderly, who are an integral part of the staffing, receive training, health assessments, and free meals.

The teen mothers are eligible for job training, health care, parenting training, and counseling. For their children, the program encompasses education, health, nutrition, and a safe, nurturing environment.

A sliding scale fee was developed by the State Health and Human Services Finance Commission which places the cost to young mothers as low as one dollar per week or as much as $40 per week, depending on the ability to pay. At least two-thirds of the population at the center are from AFDC/income-eligible families.

Extra Needs of Teens and Their Children

Several caregivers in day care centers catering both to children with teen parents and those with older parents commented on the extra needs of the teen parents and their children. This may seem overwhelming to day care workers. A lot of energy may be needed for working not only with the babies, but also with the teen parents.

Many teen parents are still adolescents and may have the erratic behavior typical of this developmental stage. A day care provider may exclaim, after a particularly trying encounter with a young mother, "She's acting just like a teenager!" At fifteen, she probably is.

Carlsbad AWARE's Van Cleave commented:

It takes extra effort to work with teen parents because they're still kids. I have to remind the staff, "Look, she's only fifteen."

It's so easy for people to think that, because she's a mother, she should be mature, but it doesn't work that way. They don't act responsible all the time.

You can observe their children and make recommendations, but they aren't going to listen unless they want to listen. You do the best you can.

It's important to help them understand how little you can expect from a baby in return for your love and your care. Most kids probably think they'll get so much from this baby immediately, and of course they're in for a rude awakening.

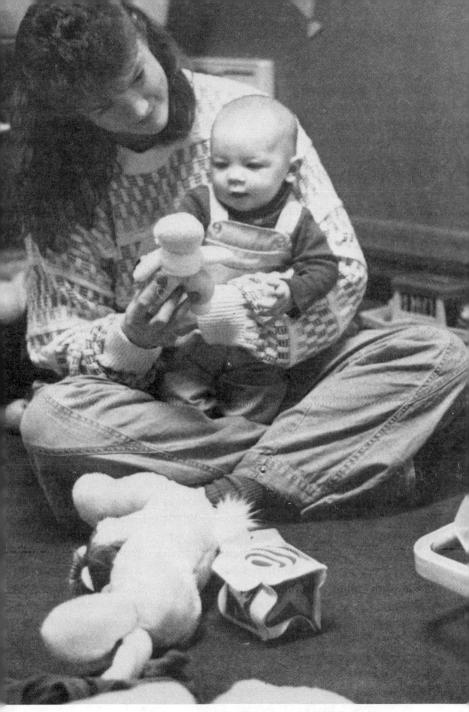

Addison County Parent-Child Center, Middlebury, Vermont

The problem is that day care providers may not be equipped to deal with adolescents and their special needs. Training on adolescent lifestyle and developmental issues is crucial for the child care staff.

Flexibility Is the Key

The Carlsbad AWARE Program operates a licensed nursery for junior and senior high school students' babies. Rooms for the nursery are provided by the school district.

Students attend their home school during the morning, and are bused to the AWARE site for afternoon classes. AWARE also provides a play group for children over two. Van Cleave explained:

> *The children can stay with us as long as their mothers attend high (or junior high) school. At first we had only the nursery for babies under two, but if the mother delivered while she was in eighth or ninth grade, she needed more than two years to finish high school. We realized care during the first two years wasn't enough.*
>
> *About one-third of the mothers seem able to cope without special services after they deliver. They return to their home school.*
>
> *However, some can't function well in the mainstream, and they may need us until they graduate. We can't say, "Okay, you've had two years of our program. Now go back to school," and then lose her.*
>
> *We helped her have a healthy baby and learn some parenting skills, but that wasn't enough. She needed to finish high school.*
>
> *So we hired an attendant with vocational/technical education funding for our over-two group. We've enrolled as many as fifteen in this play group, but we've never had more than eight attending at once.*
>
> *Some of our eighth and ninth graders stay with us all day. Some of their families object to their being mainstreamed, and for some, it's either stay here or drop out. Flexibility is the key.*

Van Cleave commented on several advantages of having child care on campus:

> *I think it's extremely important for the young mothers to work in the nursery. In addition to learning parenting, working there gives them a sense of responsibility to the program. Nursery staff are good role models, and this helps the young mothers become better parents.*
>
> *We think the babies get a tremendous start in life by being with other children during this stage.*
>
> *We hit heavily on birth control. We keep saying having another baby would limit their future so much. There were four years when no one in our program had a second baby within a year after the first, and the other three years, only five percent were pregnant again within a year.*

Van Cleave considers herself a community organizer, and boasts of the strong local support for AWARE. Community people are regularly scheduled by staff to talk to AWARE students about their jobs and the resources they can offer the young mothers. "We don't want anyone to leave our program without knowing everything this community can offer them, both now and when their children are older," Van Cleave stressed.

Van Cleave's emphasis on input from community resources for young parents should be an important part of any program serving young parents. Seldom, if ever, does a community have all the necessary resources to meet the many needs of its young parents. Even those resources that are available, however, may go unused because young parents either don't know about them, or are unable to access the services without help.

The case management approach is especially crucial here. Having one helping person responsible for assisting each young parent in meeting her health, social and education needs, whether through referrals or on-site provision, usually means a much higher percentage of young parents will utilize the services they need so desperately.

Issues to Consider

Community attitudes may be punitive and judgmental. If you provide child care, you may be accused of "making things too easy for those girls." People may feel providing child care at the school will be an incentive for other students to get pregnant. In reality, child care on campus (complete with crying babies, dirty diapers, and constant work) may help non-parents understand better the difficulties inherent in caring for little children.

You may hear that schools aren't in the social service business. But schools *are* in the business of educating young people. Child care for students' children may be a crucial aspect of providing that education.

Communities need to be reminded frequently that support services including child care can reduce repeat pregnancies, provide critical parenting education, and make it possible for young parents to become job-ready.

Joyce Keller Huff, Coordinator, **Marshalltown High School Teen Parent Program, Marshalltown, Iowa,** explained her approach to getting support for a child care program for student parents at her school:

> *We need to talk about the benefits of working with that two-week old child. That's the approach I used in selling the child care idea because our principal wasn't sold on this part at all. I said, "You realize these children will be in school in five years. We'll be getting them back and they won't be babies then. We need to help those babies get a good start **now**." That's when he decided intervention was a good idea.*

Child care for the Marshalltown program participants' babies is provided through day care homes, and is funded through Vocational Home Economics. Huff gets lists of day care homes in school neighborhoods, then coordinates placement of the young parents' babies.

Project Redirection, El Paso, Texas, relies to a great extent on day care homes for their students' children, according to Carol Wilder, Director. She commented:

*We considered putting more day care in our high
schools. At first I thought that would be great, and easier
for the girls. But unless the school provides the transportation, and they don't here, I'm not sure it would be much
easier.*

*Besides, day care is real life. It's part of learning to be
self-sufficient and part of being a parent—taking the baby
to the day care home. We find our students develop good
relationships with the day care people.*

Project Redirection has a staff member in charge of contract-
ing with day care homes and helping young mothers with the
placement of their babies. This person also monitors the homes
through visits to see that the quality of care is optimal, according
to Wilder.

Setting Standards for Child Care

Teen Renaissance, the high school program for pregnant and
parenting teens in **Brighton, Colorado,** had an infant center on
campus for several years. This center was the focus of parenting
education, and was designed as a child development center,
working with parents to provide individualized and appropriate
activities for each child.

However, several years ago the center was closed, and the
district contracted with a community day care facility to provide
care for the students' children.

Teacher Sue Dolezal commented:

*Theoretically, this was an exciting and appropriate
change. However, we had had a model child development/
parenting center, and when we switched to contract day
care, we lost control.*

*When we discovered the children were spending too
much time in their cribs and that not many activities were
provided for them, we decided we needed to set some
standards for the care of our babies.*

*We also asked the mothers to encourage better care of
their children by choosing three activities each wanted her*

child to work on. The mother then asks the day care
workers to practice those activities with her child.

Now through their advisory committee, Teen Renaissance is
developing standards for day care and child development for
children of teen parents. "We'll probably continue to contract
with this day care facility, but we're going to put more provi-
sions in the contract concerned with optimal standards for child
development," Dolezal explained. She continued:

> *We asked the director of the day care center and a*
> *child development specialist from the local university to*
> *be on the committee along with our regular advisory*
> *committee members. People from our committee visit the*
> *center once a week.*
> *Having the day care director involved with our com-*
> *mittee is helping her understand the special needs of teen*
> *mothers and their children. I think the service is*
> *improving.*

Dolezal's experience pinpoints the need to monitor child care
services used by schoolage parents. Young parents also should
be encouraged to monitor closely the care their children receive
from others.

Need Seems Endless

If a school district provides sensitive counseling plus a
variety of excellent special services for pregnant teenagers, they
may succeed in keeping these young people in school *until their
babies are born*. After childbirth, however, many young mothers
need more expensive help from the school. Those who keep
their babies to rear themselves obviously cannot attend school
unless they have child care. In many families, no one is available to help with this service.

A good developmental child care center on campus offers
several distinct advantages. First, of course, it makes it possible
for young mothers to continue their education and to obtain job
skills so they can become productive citizens.

Second, working in the Center with her own child and taking the parenting class which should be an integral part of the program helps young parents learn the parenting skills so important for their children's optimal development.

Third, the babies and toddlers in a good developmental center are generally ahead of their stay-at-home peers in social, emotional, and intellectual development. Ilustrating this concept are a number of research projects which have focused on the long-term benefits to children who received high-quality day care during their early years.

But good developmental child care is expensive, and few school districts provide it. When money is scarce, it is difficult for a district to be far-sighted enough to provide the funding now for projects which may not show cost-savings for several years.

If your district does not provide a child care center for students' children, do all you can to start a center. In the meantime, are family day care services available in the vicinity of your schools? Perhaps school personnel or a community group can provide leadership in making these services available to school-age parents. Funding might be available through job training programs or a local business or philanthropic group.

The need for child care in many areas seems endless, and most programs have waiting lists.

In some schools the young mother is allowed to take her baby to class with her during the first few months. This can be frustrating for student and teachers, but it can also enhance the bonding between mother and baby as well as allowing the young mother to continue school.

Teen fathers should, of course, be involved in parenting activities and responsibilities as much as teen mothers. If he is available, he should be strongly encouraged to participate. A male staff member can be an asset in attracting young men into the program.

Documenting the success of child care programs is essential. We generally don't have adequate data on the numbers of teens who leave school because of pregnancy, and who do not return to school because of lack of child care.

We need to gather that data, but we also need to show the results for those teens who do stay in school after childbirth. How many graduate? Do they get jobs? If you provide child care for school-age parents, can you show less dependency on welfare because of the support provided by the child care center?

What about the children? Through follow-up study, you may be able to show less need for Special Education services several years later for children enrolled in the school's infant center during their early years.

Payoff Is High

Providing a developmental child care center for students' babies and toddlers is, in the long run, truly cost-effective. Young parents who are able to continue their education and become job-ready will soon repay to society, through their taxes, the cost of the child care services which made their continued education possible. Without child care, a high percentage of these young mothers must depend on welfare for support. A fiscally conservative community should respond quickly to the needs of these young parents.

Providing for the needs of teenage parents and their children is a formidable task, but one with multiple payoffs. If teenage parents continue their education and are helped to become adequate and loving parents, everybody wins—the teenagers themselves, their babies, and society.

The price for providing these services is high. The price for not providing them is far higher.

CHAPTER 11

Developing
A Community Coalition

A coalition is a group of individuals or organizations that come together around a common concern or issue. Most of the people and programs described in this book are part of a wider community, state, and/or national coalition of people concerned with the adolescent pregnancy prevention continuum.

In establishing your program, you have, no doubt, contacted a network of people throughout your community who are also interested in these issues. You've contacted organizations that are providing programs all along the adolescent pregnancy prevention continuum. Bringing these individual and organizational resources together as a network or coalition can be advantageous for all of you.

Coalitions come in all sizes, shapes and structures. They are most effective when they have a clear purpose, a well-defined (but not necessarily complex) structure, and ownership in the collective goal. Collaborative activities can involve a very informal network of people who meet together to share information. They can also be highly structured efforts that are focused on a specific issue with a specific action plan.

Why a Coalition?

In determining who might join a coalition, think about which populations are most likely to be interested in the group's goals and issues. What motivation can be provided to get these persons to join the effort? What steps should be taken to achieve balanced participation from all segments of the community?

Actually, every group in the community has a role to play in addressing adolescent pregnancy:

- **Schools** are where most of the young people are.
- **Health care facilities** promote health and wellness.
- **Voluntary organizations** initiate service projects.
- **United Way** sets funding priorities and raises funds to underwrite the delivery of services to meet human needs.
- **Local government** is concerned about public costs related to adolescent pregnancy.
- **Business** wants a skilled labor force which means young people completing their education.
- **Religious community** serves the needs of young people and their families.
- **Youth-serving agencies** are concerned about meeting the needs of youth.
- **Parents** want their children to grow into adulthood with hopeful, healthy futures.
- **Community foundations** are interested in funding programs that make a difference in the quality of life in the community.

Without some mechanism to communicate information and coordinate activities, valuable time and resources can be wasted with duplication in some areas and major gaps in services in others. Coalitions allow a diversity of people to participate which can more accurately reflect the composition and values of the total community. Coalitions also offer an opportunity to develop a more coordinated, comprehensive service delivery system so young people not served in one program can be referred to a program that will meet their unique needs.

What a Coalition Can Do

There are a number of roles a local coalition may assume. All of them are important in building a climate that makes adolescent pregnancy prevention a priority.

These roles include:

- **Public awareness** and information;
- **Coordination** of resource-sharing opportunities;
- **Training/technical assistance** for program providers;
- **Information and advice** for decision-makers and local officials related to the needs of adolescents, and program and policies to meet the needs;
- **Monitoring** programs, services, and policies;
- **Advocacy network;**
- **Initiation** of special projects or activities;
- **Catalyst** for program and policy development.

The major role at the beginning of a coalition's existence is often directed at increasing community awareness. This involves helping the community "discover" that they have a problem that needs to be addressed. That is important for building interest in and support for the coalition and its future activities.

Broad Representation Essential

Concerned community citizens, as individuals or as representatives of existing groups, should be encouraged to take the initiative in mobilizing community teen pregnancy coalitions. The catalyst for a coalition can come from any number of areas, not just from a person or program directly dealing with adolescent pregnancy on a daily basis.

The group needs to have broad representation from the start, drawing from youth agencies, local government, the school system, health agencies, business and corporate sector, media, volunteer organizations, legal system, religious groups, PTAs, community groups, and teens themselves. Each group brings a particular perspective and different resources to the issue.

Toni Brown, past president of NOAPP, stressed that broad-based representation from all segments of the community is crucial to the success of a local adolescent pregnancy coalition. She commented:

Volunteers from a variety of backgrounds and experience will reflect the value system of the community. You need to have different points of view represented on a coalition so the conclusions they reach are valid in the eyes of the community.

Coalitions need to be careful to have more community volunteers than direct service providers represented on the group. As knowledgeable as the service providers are, they need to give the community volunteers time to discover the scope of the problem and determine what might be done to address it. This builds ownership in the process and in the eventual programs. If the coalition becomes too heavily represented by service providers, you soon may slip back to square one.

You must always continue to educate the power-brokers. This is an on-going process as the power-brokers will change over time. They make things happen in the community, and you need their support.

Who Should Participate?

The **North Carolina Coalition on Adolescent Pregnancy (NCCAP)** developed a list of groups to consider contacting when establishing a local coalition:

- Schools
- Parents
- Neighborhood/Volunteer groups
- Agencies
- Health care
- Media
- Business
- Legal/Government
- Church
- Peers

Barbara Huberman, Executive Director of NCCAP, described NCCAP's beginning:

We started with a planning group which met for six months trying to get things going. It seemed to dwell on the complexity of the problems, the lack of resources, and other negatives until we were immobilized. At that point, a few key members of the group decided they were tired of being part of an "Ain't It Awful Club," and got things moving.

First, we defined what we wanted the coalition to be in the community—an advocate, a catalyst, a facilitator, a coordinator—the group that would create on-going awareness of the problem. We started the coalition by holding a community forum. We defined ten major areas (see above) that we wanted to target to involve people. These areas became ten task forces. We assigned a facilitator to each task force area, and they were responsible for getting fifteen people to participate in the forum.

More than two hundred people attended the day-long meeting. The morning was spent giving basic information, creating awareness, and defining a basic plan of action. In the afternoon, the participants divided into the task forces and brainstormed to develop a wish list of things that could be done in the community, from that issue perspective, to promote adolescent pregnancy prevention.

Commitment cards were distributed to determine who was interested in being involved, and in what ways. From those response cards, we identified our leadership and built our board of directors. The task force information served as the basis for the development of the goals and objectives and for our first grant. We received enough funding from our initial grant proposal to enable us to hire a director on a part-time basis.

Having so many different groups involved from the beginning helped us secure a lot of in-kind resources. The school system donated paper and printing; the community college provided office space and a phone.

Organizing a Coalition

The National Organization on Adolescent Pregnancy and Parenting has highlighted ten key issues to consider when building a community coalition:

1) **Create Awareness/Identify Interest.** Are people aware of teen pregnancy and its impact in your community? Do they truly understand both the human and economic costs? Does each segment of the community understand the impact of adolescent pregnancy on them, their work, and their lives?

2) **Establish entity and determine membership.** What are your boundaries? Where is your natural base of support? Whose authorization or approval does the coalition need to gain support? What individuals and groups might have an interest in the issue? Is there a balance between service providers and community leaders? Are all major segments of the community represented?

3) **Identify leadership.** Who are the people who make decisions and make things happen in the community—people who have clout, contacts, and access to resources? How will a chairperson be selected to facilitate meetings and activities, designate responsibility, and oversee the group's coordination of efforts?

4) **Define your mission and purpose.** What is your vision? What are the desired outcomes you would like to see achieved in your community? What role will the coalition play in directing and coordinating efforts toward the realization of the vision and desired outcomes?

5) **Determine structure.** What are the lines of accountability? How will the various participants in the coalition relate to each other? In what way will the leadership be identified? What are the expectations of the leadership and the participants? Will formal bylaws be established? Will committees or task forces be needed to carry out the work of the coalition?

6) **Develop the process.** How will the coalition work and get things done? Who will do what? What are the organizational guidelines and procedures? How often will the coalition meet? How will the meetings and events be planned and carried out?

7) **Collect data and do homework.** Does the coalition have the basic information to develop its goals and plan of work? Is

the data clear, concise, and useable? What are the real
needs in the community that the coalition might address?

8) **Develop a plan and goals.** What are the goals, objectives,
and activities or events that the coalition will pursue? What
is the timetable for accomplishment? Who is responsible?
What resources will each require? What are the short-term
goals and what are the long-term goals?

9) **Develop operational support.** What will the funding base be
for the coalition? How much funding will be needed in the
short-term and long-term? How can a diversity of funding
sources be developed?

10) **Define an evaluation process.** How will the effectiveness
of the coalition be measured? Are your short-term and
long-term goals clear and realistic? How will you know if
you have achieved your desired outcomes? Who will be
responsible for evaluating the coalition's progress?

Leadership Is Critical

In any program, the leaders set the tone. For a coalition to
work well, it is important to have strong leadership that understands the delicate nature of blending the personalities, expectations, and agendas of those involved. It is also important to
rotate leadership regularly to keep the organization dynamic.

You need to have organizational representatives on the
coalition who are at a high enough level within the organization
to make decisions or to get the decisions made in a short time
frame. Otherwise, the coalition efforts can become paralyzed.

It is important to recruit leadership and participants who are
really interested in the issue and want to be there. It doesn't
matter if some participants don't have contact with the issue on
a daily basis. Understanding, a willingness to learn about the
issue, and a genuine commitment can be as important to the
success of a coalition as in-depth knowledge in the field.

Many coalitions try to avoid creating "designated seats" on
their coalition—this one for the health department, that one for
the PTA. With this plan, too often, someone gets assigned to the
coalition as a part of their responsibility with the other group,
not because they really want to be part of the coalition.

Building an Identity

The coalition will want to establish a name, mailing address, and phone number to use in promoting the group. Be careful when selecting the name. It should be positive and as clear as possible. It needs to be dynamic and sound like something people would want to support and join.

Some initial funding will be needed for stationary, postage, printing, and other operational expenses. Some of these items may be provided in-kind by some of the participating groups.

Identify one or two people to be the main contacts to receive information, handle calls, and deal with correspondence. Clarify who can speak on behalf of the coalition to the media or other groups, and what the parameters of their statements might cover.

The coalition will need a regular place to meet. It's sometimes best to pick a neutral place to avoid turf struggles. The group also needs to determine how often it will meet, and the most appropriate time for the people involved. And like other groups, the coalition will need to determine what's appropriate for the coalition as a whole to discuss, and what should be handled by task forces or a steering committee.

Use the early meetings to provide information, build enthusiasm, and encourage individual commitment. People become committed only if they feel their opinions count. This requires that they become personally involved from the first meeting. Allow everyone some type of "air time," but structure the discussion so it moves forward efficiently and stays on task.

Setting the Direction

The coalition needs to identify specific goals and objectives which reflect the organizational direction of the group. Sessions to set goals can become frustrating. Brainstorm a number of ideas, and then rank them in priority order. There are several techniques for this type of activity. The important thing to remember is to let everyone participate and have ownership in the results. These goals and objectives should then be recorded, shared with all participants, and reviewed on a periodic basis.

Existing lines of communication (businesses, churches, schools, etc.) should be utilized as a cost effective means of informing the community of the activities and for recruiting new participants.

An effective adolescent pregnancy coalition should not be organized underground. Getting an endorsement (written if possible) from heads of existing organizations creates a favorable climate from the beginning. Later, agency representatives who are members of the coalition will participate more freely because they know the project is endorsed by their director.

Service Provider Networks

The type of coalition referred to in this chapter is a community-wide model that includes service providers as one of many groups to be involved. There are valid reasons, however, for having a network of service providers in the community meeting on a regular basis to discuss adolescent pregnancy issues. These groups can share information, meet with their peers, and gain a more accurate understanding of the services available for young people in the community.

Such a network also helps service providers avoid costly duplication of programs, make better referrals to other programs, and develop collaborative activities. In some areas, the service provider network may be linked as a part of a larger community-wide coalition. In other areas, it may be a totally separate entity.

For this type of network, it's preferable to rotate the meetings to different agencies, and to rotate the leadership. Part of the time during these meetings can be given to the sharing of information about upcoming activities or for brief presentations about partciular agencies or events.

The Coalition on Responsible Parenting and Adolescent Sexuality (CORPAS) in Dallas, Texas, is an example of an active service provider's network. They meet monthly, and they select a different topic focus each month. Membership is open to any agency interested, and they work together on such projects as National Family Sexuality Education Month and on information pieces and community-wide programs. Jesse Sandoval, senior consultant for Youth Service Planning, Community Council of Greater Dallas, pointed out that CORPAS is relatively low-cost to maintain from an administrative standpoint, thanks to a lot of volunteer effort on the part of the agencies involved.

Pitfalls to Avoid

Bill Milliken, founder and president of the **Cities in Schools** program, stated that too often social service collaboration has meant "bringing the wagons in a circle and shooting at each other." Sadly, that has been true in some cases. The barriers to effective coalition building can be significant.

Some local funding sources may pit agency against agency vying for funding. Turf issues and organizational issues surface. People come to the issue of adolescent pregnancy with different perspectives, agendas, and sets of priorities. Personality conflicts prove difficult in collaborative efforts. These barriers are real, but can be overcome with thought, planning, and enough flexibility to meet the needs of the individuals and organizations involved.

Frank Barry, Family Life Development Center, Department of Human Development and Family Studies, College of Human Ecology, Cornell University, Ithaca, New York, authored *Tips for the Organizer: Practical Steps in Organizing a Community Task Force*. He suggests avoiding the following pitfalls:

1) Neglecting to involve, or at least advise, key people in the community about the coalition.
2) Spending six months or more trying to define your purpose.
3) Starting a study or survey that takes a year, and prevents other decisions or actions until its completion.
4) Becoming overly preoccupied with organizational structure such as bylaws.
5) Developing beautiful plans but neglecting to assign responsibility for carrying them out.
6) Neglecting to assign deadlines, or at least setting target dates.
7) Failing to develop the ability to deal with hard issues such as group leadership and agency turfism, local conservative or liberal attitudes.
8) Turning into discussion group rather than an action group.

9) Failure to build in a process for self-evaluation.
10) Losing sight of the young people for whom the coalition exists.

Maintaining Involvement

Motivating enthusiastic and active participation in a coalition over time requires creative thought and effort.

Having ownership in the activities, feeling an integral part of the process, and recognizing the successful completion of task will give the group a sense of achievement.

A few years back, Mary Ann Liebert, President and Executive Director of the Washington Alliance Concerned with School Age Parents and president of NOAPP, and Melinda Harmon, Office of Parent and Child Health Services in Washington state (OPCH), attended a national planning conference, "Inventing the Future," sponsored by the National Organization on Adolescent Pregnancy and Parenting.

At the conference, Washington was selected by the participants from fourteen states in the western region to develop and implement a state coalition model to address the problems of adolescent pregnancy.

OPCH, a part of the Department of Social and Health Services, and WACSAP formed a public/private partnership to create a state-wide Steering Committee on Adolescent Pregnancy Prevention, Pregnancy, and Parenting. The Steering Committee was composed of seventy-five members from diverse public and private organizations. Seventeen initiative groups were established and met monthly to study specific issues and develop action plans. In total, three hundred volunteers contributed over fifteen thousand hours to the work of the Steering Committee during its first year.

Keeping that many individuals informed and actively involved was a major challenge, according to Liebert. They were asked recently why they stayed involved in the coalition. Their reasons varied:

"Commitment to the issue."

"Participation in identifying problems and generating solutions."

"Helps make an impact on a different level from my daily work."

"I can see a step-by-step approach to where we want to go."

"We're not just talking—we're doing."

Liebert maintains that, in her experience over the years, coalitions at both the local and state level have proved to be an effective means of soliciting community commitment, securing resources, and impacting services. There is more than one solution to the problems of adolescent pregnancy prevention, pregnancy, and parenting, she says, and by working collaboratively, individuals can have a greater impact on both their local communities and on state policies. Increased communication and coordination between agencies and organizations has continually led to better coordinated services.

Maintaining a strong local coalition involves understanding the individual or the agency's role in the coalition, according to Liebert:

> *This includes acknowledging how they can also benefit from the coalition while they are contributing to its success. It's important that everyone feel ownership in the process of establishing goals and objectives, to evaluate regularly, and to celebrate accomplishments verbally as well as in writing She concluded:*

> *Members need to share a vision of what they want to accomplish and strategies of how to get there. Give members points of departure at completion of task so they can feel a sense of accomplishment, and move on if they want to, or ask for time-limited recommitment. Recruit new members as needed or appropriate to fill in gaps.*

> *The key is to keep moving forward, celebrating each milestone.*

CHAPTER 12

Keeping
The Vision Alive

The wide variety of programs included in this book shows but a sampling of the many ways groups in local communities are providing successful adolescent pregnancy prevention and care activities that meet the needs of young people. They have identified a need and pulled together the resources to meet that need. And what works in Bangor, Maine, may be different than the programs that prove successful in San Antonio, Texas, or in a small community in Kansas.

Adolescence often is a difficult time for boys and girls. Simply being there, listening, and caring thus become key factors in most programs serving teens. A flyer listing programs available at The Door in New York City says it is "A place to get help. . .A place to get it together. . .A place to be together." That says a lot to teens.

Whether your vision includes a prevention or care program— start where you are. Even the large, comprehensive programs started small. The most important thing is to start *somewhere*.

Back to the Basics

Today creative program providers and community leaders are devising ways to serve the needs of the whole person. These needs include health, education, recreation, and social as well as the other less tangible needs, the spiritual and inspirational. Many of the things service providers consider important in developing programs that successfully meet the needs of young people aren't new issues. They reflect the basic strategies that programs serving youth have known and applied over the years:

- **Self-esteem** — the foundation people need in order to achieve their potential.
- **Access to a variety of services and learning experiences** — including health care, social services, education, recreation, and job-related opportunities.
- **Friendship** — peers and others
- **Caring adults** — as role models and mentors
- **A sense of belonging** — and a sense of community
- **Having personal goals** — and support in working toward those goals.
- **Positive life options** — being able to be somebody without having a baby too soon.

Self-Esteem Provides the Foundation

Improving clients' self-esteem is basic to the success of programs serving young people, especially young people at risk for early pregnancy or parenting.

The development of self-esteem starts early and stems largely from parents, teachers, family members, and other important adults in a young child's life. The quality of these relationships is an extremely important factor in the growth of the child's self-esteem.

How young people feel about themselves affects strongly the decisions they make as they move from childhood to adulthood through the precarious pathways of adolescence. Every child needs to hear the message at home, at school, and in the community: "You are loved, respected, and accepted as you are. Your ideas and feelings are taken seriously."

Timing Is the Problem

Karen Pittman, Director, Adolescent Pregnancy Prevention, Education Division, Children's Defense Fund (CDF), discussed the timing factor in adolescent pregnancy and parenthood:

Adolescents always have passed through a period of difficult, often troubled adjustment to adult life. This transition has become more complicated in recent decades, however, because our society is making greater demands on teens, and because the adverse consequences of certain teen behaviors are more severe than they used to be.

Substance abuse, sexually transmitted diseases, suicide, depression, and stress have become increasingly common among adolescents, including a growing proportion of younger teens and even some pre-teens. The rapid growth in these problems, collectively termed "the new morbidity," is cause for serious concern as the severity of related risks dictates that they cannot be considered a natural part of growing up.

Too-early parenthood and leaving high school before graduation are often interrelated with the "new morbidity" health problems. But sexual activity, pregnancy, and school-leaving differ from the health-linked problems in an important way. Unlike substance abuse or suicide, these are viewed as positive—later. Both becoming a parent and leaving school are important and expected markers of adulthood. The timing of their occurrence is crucial to the effect they have on a youth's life.

When teens become parents or leave school before they have gained the skills, credentials, and maturity needed to secure employment, raise a child, and balance the demands of adult life, they risk foreclosing many options for their own future and the future of their children.

To change teens' behavior, we must give them a sense of hope and options for the future. A teen's ultimate chance of success as an adult depends on two factors: awareness of opportunities for success in the adult world that are meaningful and likely to be available, and adequate preparation to meet the adult world's challenges.

Including the Extended Family

Mary Butcher founded **Services for Young Families, Cleveland, Ohio,** and directed the program for twenty-one years. She stressed the importance of including boyfriends/husbands and the extended family in services provided for pregnant and parenting teen women:

When a young girl has a baby, she leans heavily on her family. If she doesn't have an extended family, she has a hard time coping with her parenting responsibilities. Often, the extended family does provide that support. Other family members, and certainly the young father, are important to the life of the young mother and the child.

One of our concerns was that this baby become an integral part of that family. Sometimes we found we were teaching things at the center that the teen's mother had never heard and didn't agree with now. We figured if we could work with the extended family, we would be ahead in terms of helping that young mother. We also realized members of the extended family often had unmet needs, too, and perhaps we could be of assistance.

So we developed a Sunday program for families, and they came in droves. We had a full meal, games, and prizes, but we also had a serious discussion at each of our meetings. For example, at least once a year the topic was male sexuality, and we'd have thirty or forty men, boyfriends, fathers of the teens, uncles, whoever.

You can't run a program with the young woman only, and ignore everybody else in her life. You have to include that boyfriend and her extended family.

Guidelines for Pregnancy Prevention

Barbara Huberman, Chairperson of the North Carolina Coalition on Adolescent Pregnancy Prevention, stresses five guidelines for decreasing adolescent pregnancy:

1) Prevention strategies must be multiple and comprehensive.
2) Prevention strategies must be long term and reflect ways to change behavior as well as attitudes and values.
3) Prevention strategies must reflect the world we live in

today, not the "good old days" of yesteryear. Media influence, the changing roles of women, the different status of families, and the decline of marriage as the solution to a pregnancy must be recognized.

4) Prevention strategies that have worked in other countries can work here too, and we must not allow a small but vocal minority to impede the necessary actions that we know we must take.

5) Prevention must be a community responsibility, not just the problem of medical, education, and social service providers.

Over and over we have stressed the need for comprehensive programs. At the same time, seldom can one program provide everything its clients need. Your action plan needs to be manageable.

At the same time, multiple services must be provided in our communities in such a way that young people don't fall through the cracks as they are referred from one service to another. Multiple services can be provided by a collaboration of groups at a single site, or they can be a decentralized network of services with a case manager who serves as an advocate for each young person in accessing the services. Plans must be carefully made that will work for the young people in each community.

From Vision to Action

Vision without action is of little value, and conversely, action without vision tends not to be productive in the long run.

We need more than rhetoric today. There is too much at stake, too many young people at risk for unintended pregnancy and early parenting, and it's too costly both in terms of human costs and dollar costs.

It is imperative that each of us be deeply involved. In every community there is a need for more coordinated, comprehensive approaches in providing adolescent pregnancy prevention and care programs to meet the needs of adolescents. Remember that successful programs flourish in a wide array of settings. There is something you can do. Focus on your vision, and *act*.

Start today!

Appendix

About the Authors

Jeanne Warren Lindsay, M.A., C.H.E., and Sharon Rodine, M.Ed., have worked with young people for many years. Each speaks frequently at conferences across the country.

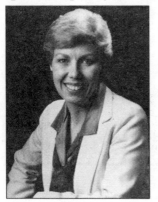

Sharon Rodine has nearly twenty years experience in leadership positions in local, state, and national organizations focused on issues of concern to women, young people, and their families. In August, 1989, she was elected president of the National Women's Political Caucus. She has served as the executive director of the National Organization on Adolescent Pregnancy and Parenting (NOAPP) for more than five years. Prior to directing the national adolescent pregnancy network, she directed the Texas Association Concerned with Adolescent Parenthood, statewide adolescent pregnancy coalition, and served as the director of the Downtown Branch, YWCA, Houston, Texas.

Sharon and her husband, Dick, have two young sons.

Jeanne founded the Teen Mother Program in the ABC Unified School District, Cerritos, California, and continues as a consultant to the program.

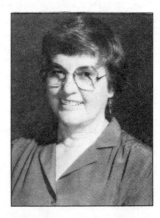

She is the author of *Teens Parenting: The Challenge of Babies and Toddlers, Pregnant Too Soon: Adoption Is an Option, Adoption Awareness: A Guide for Teachers, Counselors, Nurses and Caring Others* (co-author), and five other books dealing with single parenting, teenage marriage, and adoption. She edits the *NOAPP Network,* NOAPP's quarterly newsletter.

She and Bob have been married for thirty-eight years, and have five children.

Resource Programs
and People

Following is a list of the people and programs included in
Teen Pregnancy Challenge, Book Two: Programs for Kids.
These resources are arranged alphabetically by *program* name
followed by the name of the quoted individual.

These are the people we especially want to thank for their
wonderful help in the research for this book. We have each
talked with most of them.

Sharon Rodine, as Executive Director of NOAPP, is in
constant contact with adolescent pregnancy prevention and care
program providers throughout the United States. Jeanne Lindsay
had a wonderful time interviewing about ninety program providers in preparation for the *Teen Pregnancy Challenge* books.

The enthusiasm of these people, who care so much about
young people, and who are making a difference in the lives of
many, is inspiring and contagious. You may want to contact
some of them.

Academy for Educational Development
Elizabeth A. McGee
100 Fifth Avenue
New York, NY 10011
212/243-1110

Adolescent Family Education
Tucson Unified School District
Sherry Betts, Director
1010 East Tenth Street
Tucson, AZ 85717
602/798-2774

Adolescent Parent Prevention Program
Helen Hill, Program Director
Green County Health Care
P.O. Box 657
Snow Hill, NC 28580
919/747-5841

Adolescent Pregnancy Program Teen Outreach
Association of Junior Leagues
660 First Avenue
New York, NY 10016
212/683-1515

Adoption Information Center
Lori Obluck, Project Coordinator
1212 South 70th Street
West Allis, WI 53214
414/453-0403

American River Hospital Teen Clinic
Karen Dodge-Keys, Director
6733 Fair Oaks Boulevard #2
Carmichael, CA 95608
916/486-8336

Betsy Bergen, Associate Prof.
Human Development and Family Studies
Kansas State University
5732 Southwest 33rd
Topeka, KS 66614
913/273-2072

BETA
Judy Peterson, Director
4680 Underhill Road
Orlando, FL 32807
407/277-1942

Boulder Valley Schools Teen Parenting Program
Gloria Parmerlee-Greiner, Director
1515 Greenbriar Boulevard
Boulder, CO 80303
303/494-1006

Boys and Babies
Sharon Winkler
Presbyterian Church of the Palms
1728 Meadowood Street
Sarasota, FL 33581
813/922-7478

The Bridge
Mary Shafer, Sharon Lockwood, Co-directors
315 North University Avenue
Fargo, ND
701/241-4900

Mary Olmstead Butcher
3661 Ludgate Road
Shaker Heights, OH 44120
216/991-7974

California Department of Ed.
Ronda Simpson, Teen Pregnancy/
Teen Parent Coordinator
Alternative Education Unit
560 J Street, Room 290
Sacramento, CA 95814
916/327-2161

Capable Adolescent Mothers (CAM)
Dolores G. Martell, Ex. Director
Crossroads Programs, Inc.
P.O. Box 321
Lumberton, NJ 08048
609/267-2002

Carlsbad AWARE Program
Win Van Cleave, Director
1505 Westridge Road
Carlsbad, NM 88220
505/885-6087

Carol Cassell, Author
7129 Edwina, NE
Albuquerque, NM 87110
505/884-9068

Center for Family Life Education
Peggy Brick,
Director of Education
575 Main Street
Hackensack, NJ, 07601
201/489-1265

Center for Population Options
1012 Fourteenth Street N.W.
Suite 1200
Washington, DC 20005
202/347-5700

Center for Public Advocacy Research
Constancia Warren, Director
Adolescent Pregnancy
and Health Projects
12 West 37th Street
New York, NY 10018
212/564-9220

Chattanooga Adolescent Awareness Team (CHAAT)
Pamela Wild, Coordinator
323 High Street
Chattanooga, TN 37403
615/755-2800

Coalition on Responsible Parenting and Adolescent Sexuality (CORPAS)
Jesse Sandoval, Senior Consultant
Youth Planning Commission
Community Council of Greater Dallas
2121 Main Street, Suite 500
Dallas, TX 75201-4321
214/741-5851

Community of Caring
Joseph P. Kennedy, Jr.,
Foundation
1350 New York Avenue, N.W.,
Suite 500
Washington, DC 20005-4709
202/393-1250

Community Maternity Services
Sr. Maureen Joyce, Director
27 North Main
Albany, NY 12203
518/482-8836

Connect, A Program for Pregnant and Parenting Teens
Ann Sandven, Project Director
Teresa Arana-Wood, Case Mgr.
Terry Reilly Health Services
1515 Third Street North
Nampa, ID 83651
208/467-4431

The Corner Health Center
Joan Chesler
47 North Huron
Ypsilanti, MI 48197
313/484-3600

DARE to Be You
Marilyn Lanphier, Director,
Adolescent Health Section
Oklahoma State Dept. of Health
P.O. Box 53551
Oklahoma City, OK 73152
405/271-4476

Dunlevy-Milbank Teenage Pregnancy Prevention Program
Michael Carrera, Director
444 East 82nd Street
New York, NY 10028
212/744-0663

East End Neighborhood House
Paul Hill, Executive Director
2749 Woodhill Road
Cleveland, OH 44104
216/791-9378

Eastern Virginia Pregnancy Hotline
Ingrid Ligeon, Program Director
130 West Plume Street
Norfolk, VA 23510
804/623-9995; 1-800-552-1861

Fairbanks Counseling and Adoption Program
Cathy Mikitka
P.O. Box 1544
Fairbanks, AK 99707
907/456-4729

Family Focus—Lawndale
Gilda Ferguson-Smith, Director
3600 West Ogden Avenue
Chicago, IL 60623
312/521-3306

Family Focus/Our Place Center
Delores Holmes, Director
2010 Dewey
Evanston, IL 60201
312/475-7570

Family Learning Center
Jean Ekins, Director
Leslie Public Schools
400 Kimball
Leslie, MI 49251
517/589-9102

Family Life Education Project
Harriett Jewett, Project Educator
661 Main Street
Colusa, CA 95932
916/458-2232

Family TALKS
Ellen Peach, Co-author
28 Averill Terrace
Waterville, ME 04901
207/877-6969

**Florida Department
of Education**
John Winn, Policy Director
Office of Policy Research and
Improvement
1701 Capitol
Tallahassee, FL 32399
904/488-1611

Lois Gatchell, Consultant
5208 S. Atlanta Avenue
Tulsa, OK 74105
918/743-2915

**Girls Club of Santa Barbara
Mother/Daughter Choices**
Linda Wagner—Advocacy Press
P.O. Box 236B
Santa Barbara, CA 93102
805/962-2728

**Gordon, Sol
Author, Lecturer, Educator**
28 Heritage Court
Belmont, CA 94002
415/595-1130

GRADS Program
Gene Todd, State Supervisor
Department of Education
Vocational Home Economics
65 South Front Street, Room 912
Columbus, OH 43266-0308
614/466-3046

**Heart to Heart Program
Parents Too Soon**
Vicki McGee, Director
510 East Allen Street
Springfield, IL 62703-2318
217/522-5539

Holy Family Services
Route 1, Box 257
Weslaco, TX 78596
512/969-2538

**Home Instruction Program for
Preschool Youngsters (HIPPY)**
Miriam Westheimer, Director
National Council of Jewish
Women—Center for the Child
53 West 23rd Street
New York, NY 10010
212/645-4048

**Intergenerational Child
Development Center**
Orangeburg-Calhoun Tech. Col.
P.O. Box 1301
Orangeburg, SC 29116
803/534-8439

Inwood House—Teen Choice
Mindy Stern, Director
Community Outreach Program
320 East 82nd Street
New York, NY 10028
212/861-4400

**It's a New Life!
Teen Pregnancy Program**
Carol Heid, Director
1818 North Meade
Appleton, WI 54911
414/738-6499

Jackson-Hinds Health Center
Aaron Shirley, M.D., Director
4433 Medgar Evers Boulevard
Jackson, MS 39213
601/362-5321

**Los Angeles Unified
School District**
Jackie Goldberg, President
Board of Education
450 North Grand Avenue
Los Angeles, CA 90012
213/625-6386

Maine Young Fathers Project
Sally Brown, Director
Human Services Resource
Development
University of Southern Maine
96 Falmouth Street
Portland, ME 04103
207/780-4216

**Male Youth
Health Enhancement Project**
Andre Watson, Director
Shiloh Baptist Church
1510 Ninth Street N.W.
Washington, DC 20001
202/232-4200

MANTALK
Forsyth County Health Dept.
P.O. Box 2975
Winston-Salem, NC 27102
919/727-8172

**March of Dimes Birth Defects
Foundation (MOD)**
Anita Gallegos
Director, Community Services
Southern California MOD
502 South Verdugo Drive
Burbank, CA 91502
818/956-8565

**March of Dimes Birth Defects
Foundation (MOD)**
William R. Randolph
Deputy Director
Community Services Department
1275 Mamaroneck Avenue
White Plains, NY 10605
914/997-4461

MELD's Young Moms
Ann Ellwood, Founder
123 North Third Street
Minneapolis, MN 55401
612/332-7563

Monserrat, Catherine
4233 Montgomery N.E.
Suite 230 West
Albuquerque, NM 87109
505/438-6038

Charles Stewart Mott Foun.
Marilyn Steele
Mott Foundation Building
Flint, MI 48502-1851
313/238-5651

National Urban League
500 East 62nd Street
New York, NY 10021
212/310-9000

National Urban League
Ed Pitt, Former Director
Adolescent Male Responsibility
Program
Health and Environmental
Services Department
784 Columbus Avenue, Apt. 8-R
New York, NY 10025

New Futures School
Caroline Gaston, Principal
5400 Cutler N.E.
Albuquerque, NM 87110
505/883-5680

New Horizons
Mary Foster, Teacher
101 North Briaroaks Road
Burleson, TX 76028
817/295-6761

**New Jersey Network
for Family Life Education**
Susan N. Wilson
Executive Coordinator
Building 4087—Kilmer Campus
Rutgers University
New Brunswick, NJ 08903
609/921-2105

**New Jersey Network
on Adolescent Pregnancy**
Ann M. Wilson, Director
73 Easton Avenue
New Brunswick, NJ 08903
201/932-8636

**North Carolina Coalition
on Adolescent Pregnancy
(NCCAP)**
Barbara Huberman, Ex. Dir.
1300 Baxter, #171
Charlotte, NC 28204
704/335-1313

Parent to Parent
Winsome Hamilton, Director
St. Johnsbury, VT 05855
802/334-6744

**Parents and Adolescents Can
Talk (PACT)**
Joye Kohl, Director
Cooperative Extension Service
Taylor Hall
Montana State University
Bozeman, MT 59717
406/994-4981

Karen Pittman, Director
Adolescent Pregnancy Prevention
Education Division
Children's Defense Fund
122 C Street, N.W.
Washington, DC 20001
202/628-8787

**Planned Parenthood of
Metropolitan Washington, DC**
Wayne Pawlowski
Director of Training
1024 North Randolph Street
Arlington, VA 22201
202/483-9055

Project Alpha
National March of Dimes Birth
Defects Foundation (MOD)
1275 Mamaroneck Avenue
White Plains, NY 10605
914/428-7100

Project Redirection
Betty Dodson, Co-Founder
720 Meadowlark
El Paso, TX 79922
915/584-1412

Project Redirection—YWCA
Carol Wilder, Director
1918 Texas Street
El Paso, TX 79901
915/533-2311

PURPOSE Program
Planned Parenthood Federation
of America
810 Seventh Avenue
New York, NY 10019
212/541-7800.
Or contact your local Planned
Parenthood office for more
information.

Roosevelt Teen Health Center
Sue Imbrie
Clinic Coordinator
Roosevelt High School
6941 North Central
Portland, OR 97203
503/248-3111

**Santa Clara County
Office of Education**
Lois J. Joesten
Independent Study Teacher
Central Independent High School
590 Thornton
San Jose, CA 95128
408/286-7522

**School Based Clinic
Support Center**
Sharon Lovick, Director
5650 Kirby Drive, #203
Houston, TX 77005
713/664-7400

Six Rivers Planned Parenthood
Mike Ware
Director of Education
2316 Harrison Avenue
Eureka, CA 95501
707/442-5709

**School/Community Program
for Sexual Risk Reduction
Among Teens**
Charles Johnson
Project Coordinator
Denmark-Olar School District #2
P.O. Box 345
Denmark, SC 29042
803/793-5001

**Sex, Health and Education
(SHE) Center**
Lynn Leight, Director
12550 Biscayne Boulevard
Miami, FL 33181
305/895-5555

**St. John's Teenage Parent
Program**
Tina Juarez
Supervisor, Alternative Programs
910 East St. Johns
Austin, TX 78752
512/451-6530

St. Paul the Apostle School
Sr. Stella Maria, Principal
1536 Selby Avenue
Los Angeles, CA 90024
213/474-1587

**Teen Age Pregnancy and
Parenting Project (TAPP)**
Amy Loomis, Director
1325 Florida Street
San Francisco, CA 94110
415/648-8810

Teen Outreach Program
Association of Junior Leagues
660 First Avenue
New York, NY 10016-3241
212/683-1515

Teen Parent Program
Joyce Keller Huff, Coordinator
Marshalltown High School
1602 South Second Avenue
Marshalltown, IA 50158
515/752-9599

**Teen Pregnancy
and Parenting Program**
Helen Guisler, Social Worker
TIV II, Road 1, Box 70-A
McVeytown, PA 17051
814/542-2501

Teen Renaissance
Sue Dolezal, Teacher
607 South Joplin Street
Aurora, CO 80017
303/659-4830

Teen Services Program
Marie E. Mitchell
Grady Memorial Hospital
80 Butler St., S.E.
Atlanta, GA 30335
404/222-2302

Teen Up
Beth Harris Brandes
Catawba County Department of
Social Services
P.O. Box 669
Newton, NC 28658
704/324-9940

Teen Age Parent Program
Georgia Chaffee, Principal
Jefferson County Public Schools
1100 Sylvia
Louisville, KY 40217
502/473-8245

Teens 'N Touch
Donald Bowan
Vice President, Program
Charlotte-Mecklenburg Urban
League, Inc.
401 East Second Street
A.M.E. Zion Building
Charlotte, NC 28202
704/376-9834

Tiospaye Teca
Rural America Initiatives
Anne Floden, Executive Director
Rural Route 1, Box 1845
Rapid City, SD 57702
605/348-9924

**Tracy High School
Infant Center**
Sally McCullough
Former Head Teacher
2202 Buenos Aires Drive
West Covina, CA 91790
818/966-4938

Urban League of Albany
Gene Swanston, Ex. Director
94 Livingston Avenue
Albany, NY 12207
518/463-3121

**Urban Middle Schools
Adolescent Pregnancy
Prevention Program**
Michele A. Cahill
School and Community Services
Academy for Educational Dev.
100 Fifth Avenue
New York, NY 10011
212/243-1110

**Washington Alliance
Concerned with School Age
Parents (WACSAP)**
Mary Ann Liebert, Ex. Director
2366 Eastlake Avenue East, #408
Seattle, WA 98102
206-323-3926

**Vivian E. Washington
Group Home**
1504 Madison Avenue
Baltimore, MD 21217
301/234-2553

**Pamela Wilson, Sexuality
Education Consultant**
4105 19th Avenue
Temple Hills, MD 20748
301/630-5587

West Dallas Youth Clinic
Truman Thomas
Executive Director, Impact, Inc.
(Former Youth Clinic Director)
2121 Main Street, Suite 500
Dallas, TX 75201-4321
214/741-585

Young Men's Clinic
Bruce Armstrong, Assistant
Clinical Professor
Center for Population
and Family Health
Columbia University
60 Haven Avenue, B-3
New York, NY 10032
212/305-6960

**Young Mothers Program—
Blackfeet Reservation**
Janet Guardipee, Teacher
Box 618
Browning High School - S.D. #9
Browning, MT 59417
406/338-215, x 251

YWCA Teen Parent Program
768 State Street
Salem, OR 97301
503/581-9922

State Contacts

Prepared by the National Organization on Adolescent Pregnancy and Parenting (NOAPP). For additional state coalition/network information, contact NOAPP, P.O. Box 2365, Reston, VA 22090. 703/435-3948.

If the state has a state coalition, it is listed. If there is no formal coalition, one of the key contacts within the state is identified.

ALABAMA — Alabama Council on Adolescent Pregnancy (ACAP), Jimmy Jacobs, Counseling and Career Guidance Section
Alabama Department of Education,
1020 Monticello Court, Montgomery, AL 36117
205/261-5241

ALASKA — Governor's Commission on Children and Youth
c/o Peter Scales, Director
Anchorage Center for Families
3745 Community Park Loop #201
Anchorage, AK 99508
907/279-0551

Helen Mehrkens
Department of Education
Educational Program Services
P.O. Box F
Juneau, AK 99811
907/465-2830

Wendy Thon
Department of Health and Social Services
1231 Gambell Street
Anchorage, AK 99501
907/274-7626

ARIZONA — Judy Walruff
Arizona Council on School Age Parenting
Governor's Office for Children
1645 West Jefferson, Suite 420
Phoenix, AZ 85007
602/542-3191

ARKANSAS — Georganne Lewis
Division of Children and Family Services
Department of Health
P.O. Box 5791
North Little Rock, AR 72119
501/372-2755

CALIFORNIA — Cynthia Scheinberg
California Alliance Concerned with School Age Parents (CACSAP)
1440 East First Street, #309
Santa Ana, CA 92701
714/972-4859

Ronda Simpson,
California Department of Education
721 Capitol Mall
P.O. Box 944272
Sacramento, CA 94244-2720
916/324-9605

COLORADO — Jan Thomas
Colorado Organization on Adolescent Pregnancy and Parenting
(COAPP)
P.O. Box 441011
Aurora, CO 80012
303/871-8248

Deborah Gilboy
Governor's Initiative on Teen Pregnancy
511 Sixteenth Street, Suite 700
Denver, CO 80202
303/825-1533

CONNECTICUT — Lorna Murphy, Executive Assistant
Department of Human Resources
1049 Asylum Avenue
Hartford, CT 06105-2431
203/566-1380

DELAWARE — Lucille Siegel
Director, Adolescent Health Services,
Department of Health and Social Services
Robbins Building — 802 Silver Lake Boulevard and Walker Road
Dover, DE 19901
302/736-4787

Sarah Bell, Vocational Education
Department of Public Instruction
P.O. Box 1402, Townsend Building
Dover, DE 19903
302/736-4681

FLORIDA — John Winn
Prevention Center, Department of Education
1701 Capitol
Tallahassee, FL 32399
904/488-1611

GEORGIA — Marie E. Mitchell
Georgia Alliance on Adolescent Pregnancy (GAAP)
80 Butler Street S.E.
Atlanta, GA 30335
404/222-2302

HAWAII — Nicola Miller
Adolescent Network, Department of Health
741-A Sunset Avenue
Honolulu, HI 96816
808/735-8427

IDAHO — David Reese
Adolescent Single Parent Committee
S.W. District Health Department
920 Main, Caldwell, ID 83605
208/459-0744

Susan Ault
Department of Health and Welfare — MCH
450 West State Street
Boise, ID 83720
208/334-5959

ILLINOIS — Jenny Knauss
Illinois Caucus on Teen Pregnancy (ICTP)
100 West Randolph, Room 6-248
Chicago, IL 60601
312/621-0021

INDIANA — Sally Goss
Indiana Council on Adolescent Pregnancy (ICAP)
Indiana Board of Health
P.O. Box 1964
Indianapolis, IN 46206-1964
317/633-0290

IOWA — Sharon Dozier
Iowa Committee on Adolescent Pregnancy (ICAP)
Department of Health, Lucas State Office Building
Des Moines, IA 50319-0075
515/281-4907

KANSAS — Jo Bryant
Kansas Action for Children
701 S.W. Jackson
Topeka, KS 66601
913/232-0550

KENTUCKY — Georgia Chaffee
Kentucky Coalition on Teen Pregnancy (KCTP)
1100 Sylvia, Louisville, KY 40217
502/454-8245

LOUISIANA — Joan Smith
Louisiana Adolescent Pregnancy Prevention Commission
Department of Health/Office of Public Health
P.O. Box 60630
New Orleans, LA 70160
504/568-5330

MAINE — Margaret Clark
Adolescent Pregnancy Coalition
74 Winthrop
Augusta, ME 04330
207/622-5188

MARYLAND — Bronwyn Mayden
Governor's Council on Adolescent Pregnancy
311 West Saratoga Street, #260
Baltimore, MD 21201
301/333-0270

MASSACHUSETTS — Joan Tighe
Alliance for Young Families
818 Harrison Avenue
Boston, MA 02118
617/482-9122

MICHIGAN — Kay Wade
Michigan Association Concerned with School Age Parents (MACSAP)
2120 Fulmer Court
Ann Arbor, MI 48103
313/482-2870, x 262

Kathleen Fojtik, NOAPP/Michigan Project
Student-Parent Center
920 Miller
Ann Arbor, MI 48103
313/994-2018

MINNESOTA — Mabel Huber
Department of Human Services
444 Lafayette Road
St. Paul, MN 55155-3832
612/296-2279

MISSISSIPPI — Sandy Maxwell
Commission on Children and Youth
301 West Pearl
Jackson, MS 39203-3093
601/949-2023

MISSOURI — Debbie Murphy
Early Childhood Education
Department of Education
P.O. Box 480
Jefferson City, MO 65102
314/751-3078

MONTANA — Marge Eliason
Services for Young Families
2611 Beech Avenue
Billings, MT 59102
406/245-7328

Elizabeth Bozdog
Montana Healthy Mothers, Healthy Babies Coalition
Adolescent Pregnancy Prevention Project
P.O. Box 876
Helena, MT 59624
406/449-8611

NEBRASKA — Barbara Pearson
Teen Pregnancy Task Force
Governor's Health Planning Coordinating Council
Department of Health
P.O. Box 95007
Lincoln, NE 68509-5007
402/471-2101

NEVADA — Pam Garten
Department of Social Services
Nevada State Welfare Division
Capitol Complex
Carson City, NV 89710
702/885-4967

NEW HAMPSHIRE — June Wood
Bureau of Maternal and Child Health
Division of Public Health
Department of Health and Human Services
6 Hazen Drive
Concord, NH 03031
603/271-4520

NEW JERSEY — Ann M. Wilson
New Jersey Network on Adolescent Pregnancy (NJNAP)
73 Easton Avenue
New Brunswick, NJ 08903
201/932-8636

NEW MEXICO — Mary Mokler
New Mexico Organization on Adolescent Pregnancy and Parenting
(NMOAPP)
P.O. Box 35997
Albuquerque, NM 87176-5997
505/299-7610

NEW YORK — State: Jim Engle, Executive Director
New York Adolescent Pregnancy Council
404 Oak Street, #206
Syracuse, NY 13202.
315/471-0564

New York City; Suzanne Hanchett
Adolescent Pregnancy and Parenting Services
Office of the Mayor
250 Broadway, #1400
New York, NY 10007
212/566-3450

NORTH CAROLINA — Barbara Huberman
North Carolina Coalition on Adolescent Pregnancy (NCCAP)
1300 Baxter, #171
Charlotte, NC 28204.
704/335-1313

NORTH DAKOTA — Virginia Peterson
Department of Education
State Capitol Building
Bismarck, ND 58505.
701/224-2316

OHIO — Wanda Harewood-Jones
Department of Education
65 S. Front Street, Room 719
Columbus, OH 43266-0308
614/466-9221

OKLAHOMA — Dot Danel
Oklahoma State University
137 Home Economics West
Stillwater, OK 74078
405/744-6570

Marilyn Lanphier, RN, MPH
Department of Health-MCH
P.O. Box 53551
Oklahoma City, OK 73152
405/271-4476

OREGON — Diane Turner
Oregon Teen Pregnancy Task Force (OTPTF)
1811 N.E. 39th Street
Portland, OR 97212
503/281-5366

PENNSYLVANIA — Gary Ledebur
Bureau of Basic Education
Student Support Services, Department of Education
333 Market Street-Fifth Floor
Harrisburg, PA 17126-0333
717/787-3755

RHODE ISLAND — Linda Nightingale Greenwood
Vocational and Adult Education
Department of Education
22 Hayes Street
Providence, RI 02908
401/277-2705

SOUTH CAROLINA — Judy Richards
Office of Vocational Education
700 Governor's Drive
Pierre, SD 57501
605/773-3423

TENNESSEE — Lewis Butler
Homebound Instruction for Pregnant Students
Department of Education
100 Cordell Hull Building
Nashville, TN 37219
615/741-7454

TEXAS — Melanie Lockhart
Texas Association Concerned with School Age Parenthood (TACSAP)
P.O. Box 249
Austin, TX 78767
512/450-0456

UTAH —Ann Cheves
Department of Social Services
120 North 200 West
Salt Lake City, UT 84103
801/538-4100

VERMONT — Bill Apao
Agency of Human Service, Department of Social Welfare
103 South Main Street
Waterbury, VT 05676
802/241-2238

VIRGINIA — Martha Gilbert
Virginia Department for Children
805 East Broad Street-11th Floor
Richmond, VA 23219
804/786-5991

WASHINGTON — Mary Ann Liebert
Washington Alliance Concerned with School Age Parents (WACSAP)
2366 Eastlake Avenue E., #408
Seattle, WA 98102
206/323-3926

WEST VIRGINIA — Bobbie Adams
West Virginia Adolescent Pregnancy and Parenting Task Force
1411 Virginia Street East
Charleston, WV 25311
304/348-4007

WISCONSIN — Peggy A. Clapp
Wisconsin Alliance Concerned with School Age Parents (WACSAP)
Lady Pitts Center
820 E. Knapp, Third Floor
Milwaukee, WI 53202
414/278-0406

WYOMING — Bruce Imfeld
Department of Health and Social Services
Hathaway Office Building
Cheyenne, WY 82002
307/777-7121

Annotated
Bibliography

Following is a selected bibliography of books and other resources dealing with and useful for adolescent pregnancy prevention and care programs. Additional resources are included in the Bibliography in *Teen Pregnancy Challenge, Book One: Strategies for Change.*

We feel the following titles are especially relevant to program development at specific points on the adolescent pregnancy prevention continuum as discussed in *Teen Pregnancy Challenge, Book Two: Programs for Kids.* They deal more specifically with prevention of too-early pregnancy, prenatal care issues, and/or services for parenting teens and their children.

There is almost no duplication in the two bibliographies. Some resources, however, are appropriate for both, and you may want to check the entries in both books.

Prices, when given, are from the 1988-1989 edition of *Books in Print,* or, when not listed in that publication, were obtained directly from the publisher of the resource. If you order directly from the publisher, check first with your public library or a bookstore to learn current prices. Then add $2.00 for shipping.

Academy for Educational Development. *Urban Middle Schools Adolescent Pregnancy Prevention Program: Documentation Report.* 1989. Academy for Educational Development, 100 Fifth Avenue, New York, NY 10011. 212/243-1110. 54 pp.
Summarizes the work of pregnancy prevention projects in middle schools in eight cities across the country.

"Adolescent Abstinence: A Guide for Family Planning Professionals." Family Life Information Exchange, P.O. Box 30436, Bethesda, MD 20814. Free.
Excellent booklet to assist professionals in counseling abstinence as best (but not only) method of prevention.

Barr, Linda, and Catherine Monserrat. *Teenage Pregnancy: A New Beginning.* 1987. New Futures, Inc., 5400 Cutler, NE, Albuquerque, NM 87110. Also available from Morning Glory Press, 6595 San Haroldo Way, Buena Park, CA 90620. 99 pp. spiral. $10.
Classic prenatal health book written especially for pregnant teenagers. Fifth grade reading level, study guide. Useful for independent study as well as in groups.

_____. *Working with Childbearing Adolescents: A Guide for Use with Teenage Pregnancy, A New Beginning.* 1986. New Futures, Inc. Also available from Morning Glory Press. 159 pp. spiral. $12.95.
Excellent guidelines for professionals working with pregnant and parenting teens.

Beckstein, Douglas. *1987 Annotated Guide to Men's Sexual and Reproductive Health Resources.* 1987. Men's Reproductive Health, P.O. Box 661, Capitola, CA 95010. 40 pp. $25.
Contains very comprehensive collection of men's reproductive health materials. Includes 627 annotations from 205 organizations. First published in 1978.

Bell, Ruth, and Leni Wildflower. *Talking with Your Teenager: A Book for Parents.* 1984. Random House, New York, NY. 150 pp. $8.95.
A thoughtful book for anyone living with, working with, or just wanting to understand teenagers and pre-teens.

Bingham, Mindy, Lari Quinn and William P. Sheehan. *Mother Daughter Choices: A Handbook for the Coordinator.* 1988. Advocacy Press, P.O. Box 236, Department A, Santa Barbara, CA 93102. 144 pp. $7.95.
A guide to sponsoring or coordinating Mother-Daughter groups. Also see **Choices: A Teen Woman's Journal for Self Awareness and Personal Planning, Challenges: A Young Man's Journal for Self-Awareness and Personal Planning,** *$14.95 each, and* **More Choices: A Strategic Planning Guide for Mixing Career and Family,** *$15.95.*

Breen, Sharon. **"Teen Parents: An Annotated Bibliography for Teen Parents and Professionals Who Work with Them."** 1988. Middle Country Public Library, Children's Services Department, 101 Eastwood Boulevard, Centereach, NY 11720. 516/585-9393. 33 pp.
Wonderful bibliography of books including novels, films, articles, and pamphlets.

Brick, Peggy, et al. **Bodies, Birth and Babies: Sexuality Education in Early Childhood.** 1989. The Center for Family Life Education, Planned Parenthood of Bergen County, Inc., 575 Main Street, Hackensack, NJ 07601. 201/489-1265. $12.95 ppd.
Manual to help preschools integrate sexuality education into their programs. Includes workshop outlines for teachers and parents. Excellent resource.

_____ and Carolyn Cooperman. **Positive Images: A New Approach to Contraceptive Education.** 1987. The Center for Family Life Education. Planned Parenthood of Bergen County, Inc. 84 pp. $17 ppd.
Offers extremely creative approach to teaching contraception. Provides lessons which encourage conscious decision-making and integrates contraceptive use into the ideology of love, relationships, and sexuality.

_____ with Catherine Charlton, Hillary Kunins, and Steve Brown. **Teaching Safer Sex.** 1989. The Center for Family Life Education, Planned Parenthood of Bergen County, Inc. 92 pp. $22.95 ppd.
A teaching manual with fifteen complete lessons for helping people assess risk, communicate with partners, and make decisions that protect.

Cahill, Michele, J. Lynne White, David Lowe, and Lauren E. Jacobs. *In School Together: School-based Child Care Serving Student Mothers.* 1987. School Services Division, Academy for Educational Development, 680 Fifth Avenue, New York, NY 10019. 135 pp. $15.
Practical how-to guide for creating school-based child care centers for students' children. Covers all phases of program development process including support strategies, staffing, program and policies, funding, and evaluation.

Campbell, Patty. *Sex Guides: Books and Films About Sexuality for Young Adults.* 1986. Garland Publishing, 136 Madison Avenue, New York, NY 10016. 374 pp. $27.
Entertaining and informative look at sex guides for young people, guides published in the United States since 1892. Analyzing sex manuals for our young people is a fascinating way of looking at changes in our culture during the past century. Includes relevant fiction titles.

Carrera, Michael. *Sexual Health for Men: Your A to Z Guide.* 1989: Michael Friedman Publishing Group, 15 West 26th, New York, NY 10010. 212/685-6610. 75 pp. $4.95.
Comprehensive listings regarding men's sexuality and sexual expression as a means of enhancing sexual literacy.

_____. *Sexual Health for Women: Your A to Z Guide.* 1989. Michael Friedman Publishing Group. 90 pp. $6.95.
Comprehensive listings regarding women's sexuality and sexual expresssion.

Carrera, Michael, Ph.D., and Julie Spain, Ph.D. *Carrera/Spain Adolescent Sexuality Report.* Carrera/Spain, Inc., P.O. Box 3000, Dept. CS, Denville, NJ 07834. $58/year.
Interesting, attractive newsletter full of good information.

Casey, Sean, and Sydney Earle Cone. *Programs at a Glance.* 1986. Center for Population Options, 1012 14th Street, N.W., Suite 1200, Washington, DC 20005. 60 pp. $10.
Presents full-page descriptions of interesting and practical approaches to the teenage pregnancy issue.

Cassell, Carol. *Straight from the Heart: How to Talk to Your Teenagers About Love and Sex.* 1987. Simon and Schuster, Simon & Schuster Building, Rockefeller Center, 1230 Avenue of the Americas, New York, NY 10020. 255 pp. $15.95.
Excellent guide for parents and for anyone who talks with kids about issues related to sex. Purpose is to show parents how to raise sexually sane teenagers, young people free from old roles and comfortable about sex, but unwilling to rush into something they aren't prepared to handle. Well researched.

Children's Defense Fund (CDF). See Bibliography in *Teen Pregnancy Challenge, Book One: Strategies for Change.*

Compton, Nancy, Mara Duncan, and Jack Hruska. *How Schools Can Combat Student Pregnancy.* 1987. NEA Professional Library, P.O. Box 509, West Haven, CT 06516. 203/934-2669. 184 pp. $10.95.
Excellent discussion of the school's role in teenage pregnancy prevention and care—an in-depth discussion of how schools can make a difference in young people's lives by dealing with these issues rather than pretending the problems don't exist.

Contemporary Health Series. Network Publications, ETR Associates, P.O. Box 1830, Santa Cruz, CA 95061-1830. 408/438-4080. Each module, $19.95.
Entering Adulthood modules: *Living in Relationships* by Betty Hubbard, 1989, 96 pp.
Understanding Reproduction, Birth and Contraception by Clint E. Bruess and Susan J. Laing, 1989, 140 pp.
Preventing Sexually Related Disease by Betty M. Hubbard, 1989, 110 pp.
Coping with Sexual Pressures by Nancy Abbey and Elizabeth Raptis Picco, 1989, 90 pp.
Into Adolescence modules: *Enhancing Self-Esteem by Dale Zevin, 1989, 84 pp.*
Living in a Family by Jory Post, 1989, 135 pp.
A Time of Change by Catherine S. Golliher, 1989, 129 pp.
Choosing Abstinence by Dale Zevin, 1989, 85 pp.
Learning About Reproduction and Birth by Catherine S. Golliher, 1989, 150 pp.
Learning About AIDS by Jory Post and Carole McPherson, 1988, 232 pp.

*Excellent collection of curriculum modules presented in two
divisions for two age groups. **Into Adolescence** is for grades five
through eight. **Entering Adulthood** considers critical health issues
in depth for grades nine through twelve. Emphasis is on building
self-esteem, decision-making, and critical-thinking skills as the
essential foundation for healthful behavior. Module format allows
flexibility. Each module is designed to fit within a total health
curriculum or to be integrated into a variety of disciplines including
health, family living, home economics, biology, science,
psychology, physical education and social studies.*

Dryfoos, Joy G. ***Putting the Boys in the Picture.*** 1988. Network
Publications, P.O. Box 1830, Santa Cruz, CA 95061-1830. 108 pp.
Paper, $19.95.
*Focuses entirely on intervention strategies for boys to prevent teen
pregnancy. Examines model programs for making contraception
and AIDS prevention information available to teenage boys.*

Emmens, Carol. ***The Abortion Controversy.*** 1987. Julian Messner,
Simon & Schuster, Inc., Simon & Schuster Building, Rockefeller
Center, 1230 Avenue of the Americas, New York, NY 10020.
137 pp. $5.95.
*Gives a detailed and fair discussion of both sides of the abortion
issue.*

Family Life Matters. New Jersey Network for Family Life Education,
Rutgers University, Building 4087, Kilmer Campus, New Brunswick, NJ 08903. $10/year covers membership and subscription to
newsletter (three issues per year).
*New Jersey is a pioneer in the field of sex education in the schools,
and this newsletter reflects their expertise.*

Family Planning Perspectives. Published bimonthly by The Alan
Guttmacher Institute, 111 Fifth Avenue, New York, NY 10003.
212/254-5656. Personal, $28; institutional, $38.
*Wonderful source for learning about latest research on adolescent
pregnancy and prevention.*

Fennelly, Katherine. ***El Embarazo Precoz: Childbearing Among
Hispanic Teenagers in the United States.*** 1988. Columbia University Center for Population and Family Health, Columbia University,
60 Haven, New York, NY 10032. Attn: Ms. Ferguson. $5.

Provides excellent research-based information on sexual activity, pregnancy and abortion, childbearing, and birth control among Hispanic teenagers in the United States.

Foster, Sallie. *The One Girl in Ten: A Self Portrait of the Teenage Mother.* 1988. Child Welfare League of America. Order from CSSC, Inc., 300 Raritan Center Parkway, P.O. Box 7816, Edison, NJ 08818. $10.95.
The author taped interviews with 126 young mothers. Through their words, she presents a broad picture of the world of teen parenthood.

Francis, Judith, and Fern Marx. *Learning Together: A National Directory of Teen Parenting and Child Care Programs.* 1989. Publications Department, Wellesley College Center for Research on Women, Wellesley College, Wellesley, MA 02181. 617/235-0320. 220 pp. $20.
Profiles more than three hundred programs serving teen parents and their children. Illustrates range of services necessary to support young families.

Gardner, Jay. *A Difficult Decision: A Compassionate Book About Abortion.* 1986. The Crossing Press, 22-D Roache Road, P.O. Box 1048, Freedom, CA 95019. 408/722-0711. 118 pp. $6.95.
Offers options and support needed to help women and couples facing unexpected pregnancy to make a choice with which they can live. Support is given for either continuing the pregnancy or having an abortion.

Garner, Barbara. *WorkWise: A Career Awareness Course for Teen Parents.* 1989. Cambridge Community Services, 99 Bishop Richard Allen Drive, Cambridge, MA 02139. 617/876-5214. 232 pp. $35. Includes Teacher's Manual and one Student Workbook. Workbook may be reproduced.
Career exploration curriculum that guides teenagers through the process of developing career goals. Designed for teen mothers.

Glenn, H. Stephen, with Jane Nelson. *Raising Children for Success: Blueprints and Building Blocks for Developing Capable People.* 1987. Sunrise Press, Fair Oaks, CA. 210 pp. $7.95.
Good insight into the basics of helping kids grow and develop.

Gordon, Sol, Ph.D. *When Living Hurts.* 1985. Union of American
Hebrew Congregations, New York, NY. 127 pp. $8.95.
*Provides insight into working with young people troubled by severe
depression and a sense of failure.*

_____, and Judith Gordon. *Raising a Child Conservatively in a
Sexually Permissive World.* 1986. Simon and Schuster, 1230
Avenue of the Americas, New York, NY 10020. 224 pp. $7.95.
Common sense approach to sex education within the family.

Hafner, Debra. *Life Planning Education: A Strategy for Teenage
Pregnancy Prevention.* Revised 1988. Center for Population
Options, 1012 14th Street, N.W., Suite 1200, Washington, DC
20005. $35.
*Confronts the possible serious economic consequences of teenage
pregnancy by educating adolescents about the important link
between vocational and family planning.*

*Healthy Mothers, Healthy Babies Coalition: Directory of Educational
Materials.* 1985. U.S. Department of Health and Human Services,
U.S. Public Health Service. Available free of charge from the
National Maternal and Child Health Clearinghouse, 38th and R
Streets, N.W., Washington, DC 20057. 170 pp.
A directory of maternal and child educational materials.

Institute of Medicine. *Prenatal Care—Reaching Mothers, Reaching
Infants.* 1988. National Academy Press, Washington, DC. 254 pp.
$19.95.
*Report by Institute of Medicine's interdisciplinary committee to
study ways to draw more women into prenatal care early in
pregnancy and of sustaining their participation until delivery.*

*Healthy Mothers, Healthy Babies: A Compendium of Program Ideas
for Serving Low-Income Women.* 1986. Department of Health and
Human Services, U.S. Public Health Service, Health Resources and
Services Administration. Available free of charge from the National
Maternal and Child Health Clearinghouse, 38th and R Streets,
N.W., Washington, DC 20057. 168 pp.
*Contains descriptions of selected programs, summary of educa-
tional efforts and needs for educational materials, and brief review
of the literature. One section deals with teenage parents.*

Helton, Anne Stewart. *Relationships Without Violence: A Curriculum for Adolescents.* 1989. Texas Gulf Coast Chapter, March of Dimes Birth Defects Foundation, 3000 Wesleyan, Suite 100, Houston, TX 77027. 713/623-2020. Curriculum and ten-minute video. $65.
Educational curriculum designed for school-age youngsters and adolescents. Program increases awareness about the problem of battering and promotes skills for nonviolent behavior.

Hoopfer, Leah. **"Coping Skills" Series.** 1986. "Peer-Plus," $15; "Group Dynamite," $13; "High on Myself," $9; and "Careers Unlimited," $13.50. Available from Janet Olsen, MSU Extension Service, 6H Berkey Hall, East Lansing, MI 48824-1111; 517-355-0180. Also "Stress Connection," $1. Available from National 4-H Council, 7100 Connecticut Avenue, Chevy Chase, MD 20815.
Materials for adolescents presented in an interesting and highly experiential format.

Human Sexuality: Values and Choices. 1986. Search Institute, 122 West Franklin, Suite 525, Minneapolis, MN 55404. Write for brochure describing materials.
Fifteen-lesson curriculum with extensive teaching helps. Targeted to grades seven and eight.

Klinman, Debra G., and Rhiana Kohl. *Fatherhood U.S.A: The First National Guide to Programs, Services, and Resources for and About Fathers.* The Fatherhood Project at Bank Street College of Education. 1984. Garland Publishing, Inc., 136 Madison Avenue, New York, NY 10016. Paper, 320 pp. $14.95.
Contains a wealth of information about many health, education, social and supportive services for "all kinds" of fathers. Projects are described and fathers' rights organizations listed.

Kramer, Patricia. *The Dynamics of Relationships: A Prevention Program for Teens.* Revised 1987. Equal Partners, Kensington, MD 20795. Student Manual and Teacher Manual, 331 pp. plus fifty pages of lessons and activities. $29.95.
A curriculum that covers a wide range of topics of interst to teens.

Krebill, Joan, and Julie Taylor. *A Teaching Guide to Preventing Adolescent Sexual Abuse.* 1988. Network Publications, ETR Associates, P.O. 1830, Santa Cruz, CA 95061-1830. 200 pp. $29.95.

*Can help school districts and community agencies develop sexual
abuse prevention programs at the secondary level. Well organized
and supportive of both teacher and students.*

Kunjufu, Jawanza. **Countering the Conspiracy to Destroy Black Boys.**
1985. African American Images, 9204 Commercial Boulevard,
Chicago, IL 60617. 38 pp. $4.95.
*Discussion of racism as it affects African-American children,
especially males.*

Leight, Lynn. **Raising Sexually Healthy Children: A Loving Guide for
Parents, Teachers, and Care-Givers.** 1988. Rawson Associates,
Macmillan Publishing Company, 866 Third Avenue, New York,
NY 10022. 212/702-2120. 284 pp. Hardcover, $17.95.
*Provides information parents need to help children view human
sexuality as a positive life force from earliest infancy.*

Lindsay, Jeanne Warren, and Catherine Paschal Monserrat. **Adoption
Awareness: A Guide for Teachers, Counselors, Nurses and
Caring Others.** 1989. Morning Glory Press, 6595 San Haroldo
Way, Buena Park, CA 90620. 286 pp. Paper, $12.95; Cloth, $17.95.
*Provides clear, compassionate and sensible guidance for anyone
working with teenagers facing untimely pregnancy. Includes
guidelines for assisting birthparents in the classroom, in the coun-
seling setting, and in the hospital as they consider their options.*

_____, and Sharon Rodine. **Teen Pregnancy Challenge, Book One:
Strategies for Change.** 1989. Morning Glory Press. 256 pp. Pap.
$14.95; Cloth, $19.95. Two-book set (**Book Two: Programs for
Kids**), $24.95, $35.95.
*Provides guidelines for developing adolescent pregnancy preven-
tion and care programs—documenting the need, gaining community
support, funding, evaluation, and other essentials.*

_____. **Parents, Pregnant Teens and the Adoption Option: Help for
Families.** 1989. Morning Glory Press. 208 pp. Paper, $8.95; Cloth,
$13.95.
*Guidance for parents of pregnant teenagers, especially those
considering the adoption alternative. Offers practical suggestions
for providing support while encouraging the young person to take
responsibility for her decisions.*

_____. *Teens Parenting: The Challenge of Babies and Toddlers.*
1981. To be revised 1990. Morning Glory Press. 320 pp. Paper,
$9.95; cloth, $14.95.
*Step-by-step guide to the development and care of children from
birth to two years. Points out special realities of life for very young
parents.*

March of Dimes Birth Defects Foundation. 1275 Mamaroneck Avenue,
White Plains, NY 10605. 914/997-4461. Or contact local March of
Dimes chapter for current listing of materials.

March of Dimes Birth Defects Foundation. **Project Alpha Training
Kit.** 1986. March of Dimes Birth Defects Foundation, Supply
Division, 1275 Mamaroneck Avenue, White Plains, NY 10605.
Leader's Guide and Training Vidcotape, $20.
*Explores problem of teenage pregnancy from male perspective.
Unique educational project helps young men learn about their role
in responsible childbearing. Co-sponsored by Phi Alpha Fraternity
and March of Dimes.*

Marsh, Carole S. *Sex Stuff for Kids 7-17.* 1988. Gallopade Publishing
Group, Main Street, Historic Bath, NC 27808. 70 pp. Illus. Paper,
$14.95. Hardcover 3-ring binder parent/teacher edition with
page-by-page guide, $24.95.
*Offers frank, humorous, straightforward and enthusiastic look at
our lifetime of sexuality. An up-beat discussion of sex generally, and
provides effectively-written and convincing explanations of reasons
to postpone sexual intercourse through the early teen years.*

Matiella, Ana Consuelo. *La Familia and Cultural Pride.* 1988.
Network Publications, P.O. Box 1830, Santa Cruz, CA 95061-1830.
408/438-4080. Two curriculum units, 185 pp, $17.95 each, plus two
student workbooks, 96 pp, $7.95 each.
*Latino Family Life Education Curriculum Series for grades five to
eight is an innovative curriculum designed to make family life
education culturally relevant for Latino youth. Strongly affirms
Latino culture and family.*

McGee, Elizabeth A., with Susan Blank. *A Stitch in Time: Helping
Young Mothers Complete High School.* 1989. Academy for
Educational Development, 100 Fifth Avenue, New York, NY
10011. $15.

Guidelines for developing collaborative community strategies for addressing the needs of pregnant and parenting teenagers. Describes a three-step process for communities to follow to improve the ways they address the educational needs of school-age mothers.

McGee, Elizabeth A. ***Training for Transition: A Guide for Training Young Mothers in Employability Skills.*** 1985. Manpower Demonstration Research Corporation, 3 Park Avenue, New York, NY 10016. 212/532-3200. 94 pp. Spiral.
Practical, accessible handbook includes thirty-six step-by-step lessons on helping young mothers prepare for jobs.

National AIDS Information Clearinghouse. Contact NAIC, P.O. Box 6003, Rockville, MD 20850. 301/762-5111. For bulk publications, call 1-800/458-5231.
Operated by the Center for Disease Control, NAIC offers information on AIDS programs and services on a national, state and local level. Training resources and educational literature and posters are available including Public Health Service publications on AIDS.

Nelson, Mary, Editor. ***Teaching Tools, Selected Articles, Family Life Educator, Volumes I-III.*** 1985. Network Publications, 1700 Mission Street, P.O. Box 1830, Santa Cruz, CA 95060-1830. Two publications, $14.95 each.
Teaching Tools contains forty-five reproducible teaching activities. ***Selected Articles*** includes twenty-nine articles plus updates on other topics.

Nickel, Phyllis Smith, and Holly Delaney. ***Working with Teen Parents: A Survey of Promising Approaches.*** 1985. The Family Resource Coalition, 230 North Michigan Avenue, Suite 1625, Chicago, IL 60601. 312/726-4750. 140 pp.
Description of services for teen parents. Each topic includes vignettes of model program activities and methods.

NOAPP Network. Quarterly newsletter. National Organization on Adolescent Pregnancy and Parenting, Box 2365, Reston, VA 22090. 16-24 pp./issue. Included with membership: individuals, $25; organizations, $75.
Legislative, program, research, and other topics dealing with adolescent pregnancy, parenthood, and prevention. Many resource reviews.

Peterson, Lynn. **"Helping Teens Wait."** 1987. The Center for Health Training, 400 Tower Building, 1809 Seventh Avenue, Seattle, WA 98101-1316. 206/447-9538. 16 pp. $3.95.
Listing of educational materials focusing on sexual abstinence for adolescents.

Polit, Denise F. *Building Self-Sufficiency: A Guide to Vocational and Employment Services for Teenage Parents.* 1986. Humanalysis, Inc., 444 Broadway, Saratoga, NY 12866. 518/587-3994. 125 pp. $6.
Guide for designing employment-related and vocational services for teen parents.

Quackenbush, Marcia, and Mary Nelson with Kay Clark. *The AIDS Challenge: Prevention Education for Young People.* 1988. Network Publications, P.O. Box 1830, Santa Cruz, CA 95061-1830. 408/429-9822. 526 pp. $24.95.
Thirty essays covering the issues related to AIDS prevention education in community and school settings. Provides excellent overview.

_____, and Pamela Sargent. *Teaching AIDS: A Resource Guide on Acquired Immune Deficiency Syndrome.* 1988. Network Publications. 163 pp. $19.95.
Excellent resource guide designed to assist teachers, youth leaders, and health educators in integrating AIDS information into their existing courses.

_____, and Sylvia Villarreal. *"Does AIDS Hurt?" Educating Young Children About AIDS.* 1988. Network Publications. 143 pp. $14.95.
Offers teachers, parents, and others who care for and love young children basic guidelines for talking with them about AIDS. Emphasizes the use of age-appropriate responses to children's questions.

Reis, Elizabeth. *5/6 F.L.A.S.H.: Family Life and Sexual Health.* Revised 1988. Loose-leaf notebook, 216 pp. $15.00. Also *7/8 F.L.A.S.H.: Family Life and Sexual Health.* Revised 1988. 363 pp, $30. Seattle-King County Department of Public Health, Ellen Phillips-Angeles, Seventh Floor, 400 Yesler Building, Seattle, WA 98104.

Sensitively written, easy-to-use lesson plans for family living course. Includes many suggestions for working with parents.

Risk and Responsibility: Teaching Sex Education in America's Schools Today. 1989. The Alan Guttmacher Institute, 111 Fifth Avenue, New York, NY 10003. 24 pp. $3. Bulk discounts.
Important research report for anyone interested in or concerned about Family Life Education in our schools.

SBC Support Center. **"School-Based Clinics: A Guide for Advocates."** 1988. Publications Department, Center for Population Options, 1012 14th Street, N.W., Suite 1200, Washington, DC 20005. 202/347-5700. 25 pp. $2.
Background information on adolescent health, tips for handling opposition, list of organizations on record in support of school-based clinics, sample policy statements, and list of resources. Their pamphlet, "Guidelines for School-Based Clinics," outlines the framework for effective school-based clinics. $1.

Sheeran, Patrick J. **Women, Society, the State, and Abortion: A Structuralist Analysis.** 1987. Praeger Publishers, Greenwood Press, Inc., 88 Post Road West, P.O. Box 5007, Westport, CT 06881-9990. 150 pp. $32.95.
Scholarly study of the present policy on abortion in the United States, analysis of the consequences of that policy, and a history of abortion over the centuries.

School-Based Health Clinics: Legal Issues. 1988. Adolescent Health Care Project, National Center for Youth Law, 1663 Mission Street, Suite 500, San Francisco, CA 94103. 415/543-3307. 50 pp. $10.
Reviews consent, confidentiality and liability issues, including an overview of legal definitions of adolescents' rights. A special section describes federal funding programs.

Smith, Thomas J., Mary Moorhouse, and Carolyn Trist. **A Practitioner's Guide: Strategies, Programs, and Resources for Youth Employability Development.** Revised 1988. Public/Private Ventures, 399 Market Street, Philadelphia, PA 19106. 215/592-9099. 92 pp. $10.
Guide to the youth employment problem, to strategies for addressing the problem successfuly, and to current programs that are effective.

Smollar, Jacqueline, and Theodora Ooms. *Young Unwed Fathers: Research Review, Policy Dilemmas and Options.* 1987. Share Resource Center, P.O. Box 30666, Bethesda, MD 20814. 301/907-6523; 1-800-537-3788. 106 pp. $5.
Synthesizes major findings of ten working papers commissioned from researchers and program professionals and summarizes 1986 symposium on the topic.

Spain, Julie, Ph.D. *Sexual, Contraceptive, and Pregnancy Choices: Counseling Adolescents.* 1988. Gardner Press, Inc., 19 Union Square West, New York, NY 10003. 160 pp. Cloth, $26.95. Paper, $16.95 ppd.
Designed to help professionals support adolescents, through empathetic and comprehensive counseling, in successful decision-making. Focuses on skills and knowledge.

Vecchiolla, Francine J., and Penelope L. Maza. *Pregnant and Parenting Adolescents: A Study of Services.* 1989. Child Welfare League of America, Inc., 440 First Street, N.W., Suite 310, Washington, DC 20001-2085. 51 pp.
Report of study of 250 CWLA member agencies undertaken to learn what services these agencies currently provide to pregnant and parenting adolescents.

Vincent, Murray L., Ed.D., Project Director. *Reducing Unintended Adolescent Pregnancy Through School/Community Educational Interventions: A South Carolina Case Study.* 1988. Division of Health Education, Center for Health Promotion and Education, Centers for Disease Control. 40 pp.
Describes the strategies and methods used to address the teen pregnancy problem in a South Carolina county in which the pregnancy rates for teens who were exposed to the school/community-based intervention decreased by more than half compared with teens not exposed to the intervention. (See pp. 69-72 of Teen Pregnancy Challenge, Book Two, for discussion of project.)

Warren, Constancia, Ph.D. *Improving Student's Access to Health Care: School-Based Health Clinics, A Briefing Paper for Policymakers.* 1987. Center for Public Advocacy Research, Inc., 12 West 37 Street, New York, NY 10018. 212/564-9220. $10.

*Discusses the valuable role school-based health clinics can play in
meeting the health care needs of children, and about the barriers
that prevent thousands of New York State's children from getting
adequate preventive and primary care. Directed primarily to state
policy makers and legislators, and to health, education, and social
service advocates.*

Weikart, David P., et al. *Changed Lives: The Effects of the Perry Preschool Program on Youths Through Age 19.* 1984. The High/Scope
Press. 600 North River Street, Ypsilanti, MI 48197. 313/485-2000.
210 pp.
*Report of the Perry Preschool Study which started in the 1960s, and
clearly shows the value of early education.*

Wilson, Susan. **Creating Family Life Education Programs in the
Public Schools: A Guide for State Education Policymakers.** 1985.
National Association of State Boards of Education, 701 North
Fairfax Street, #304, Alexandria, VA 22314. 24 pp. $4.
*Outlines basic decisions, strategies, and obstacles State Boards of
Education must face in dealing with Family Life Education in public
schools. Includes copy of New Jersey regulation mandating family
life education.*

Index

ALSO BY JEANNE LINDSAY/SHARON RODINE:

TEEN PREGNANCY CHALLENGE, Book One:
Strategies for Change
Practical guidelines for developing adolescent pregnancy prevention
and care programs blended with poignant descriptions of the needs of
young people and the caring adults striving to meet these needs.

OTHER BOOKS BY JEANNE WARREN LINDSAY:

TEENS PARENTING: The Challenge of Babies and Toddlers
How to parent the first two years—with an emphasis on the special
needs of teenage parents.

PREGNANT TOO SOON: Adoption Is an Option
Advocates choice. Young women who were, by their own admission,
"pregnant too soon," tell their stories.

TEENAGE MARRIAGE: Coping with Reality
Gives teenagers a picture of the realities of marriage—a look at the
difficulties they may encounter if they say "I do" too soon.

TEENS LOOK AT MARRIAGE: Rainbows, Roles and Reality
Describes the research behind *Teenage Marriage*. Helps you understand
the culture of teenage couples.

ADOPTION AWARENESS: A Guide for Teachers, Nurses,
Counselors and Caring Others (with Catherine Monserrat)
A guide for anyone wishing to support the adoption alternative in crisis
pregnancy.

PARENTS, PREGNANT TEENS AND THE ADOPTION OPTION:
Help for Families
For all parents who feel alone and without support for themselves as
their daughter faces too-early pregnancy and the difficult adoption/
keeping decision.

DO I HAVE A DADDY? A Story About a Single-Parent Child
Picture/story book especially for children with only one parent. Includes
special ten-page section for single parent.

OPEN ADOPTION: A Caring Option
A fascinating and sensitive account of the new world of adoption. Read
about birthparents choosing adoptive parents for their baby and adoptive
parents maintaining contact with their baby's birthparents.

Please see ordering information on back of page.

MORNING GLORY PRESS
6595 San Haroldo Way, Buena Park, CA 90620
714/828-1998

Please send me the following:

Quantity	Title	Price	Total
	Teen Pregnancy Challenge, Book 1: Strategies for Change		
	Paper, ISBN 0930934-34-2	$14.95	————
	Cloth, ISBN 0930934-35-0	19.95	————
	Teen Pregnancy Challenge, Book 2: Programs for Kids		
	Paper, ISBN 0930934-38-5	14.95	————
	Cloth, ISBN 0930934-39-3	19.95	————
	SPECIAL—Teen Pregnancy Challenge—2-book set		
	Paper, ISBN 0930934-40-7	24.95	————
	Cloth, ISBN 0930934-41-5	34.95	————
	Teenage Parents: Coping with Three-Generation Living		
	Available spring, 1990		
	Teens Parenting: The Challenge of Babies and Toddlers		
	Paper, ISBN 0930934-06-7	9.95	————
	Pregnant Too Soon: Adoption Is an Option		
	Paper, ISBN 0930934-25-3	9.95	————
	Cloth, ISBN 0930934-26-1	15.95	————
	Adoption Awareness: A Guide for Teachers, Counselors, Nurses and Caring Others		
	Paper, ISBN 0930934-32-6	12.95	————
	Cloth, ISBN 0930934-33-4	17.95	————
	Parents, Pregnant Teens and the Adoption Option		
	Paper, ISBN 0930934-28-8	8.95	————
	Cloth, ISBN 0930934-29-6	13.95	————
	Teenage Marriage: Coping with Reality		
	Paper, ISBN 0930934-30-x	9.95	————
	Cloth, ISBN 0930934-31-8	15.95	————
	Teens Look at Marriage: Rainbows, Roles and Reality	9.95	————
	Teenage Pregnancy: A New Beginning	10.00	————
	Working with Childbearing Adolescents	12.95	————
	Do I Have a Daddy? A Story About a Single-Parent Child	3.95	————
	Open Adoption: A Caring Option	9.95	————
	TOTAL		————

Please add postage: 1-3 bks, $2; 4+, 60¢/book.

California residents add 6% sales tax.

Ask about quantity discounts, Teacher's Guides, Study Guides.   TOTAL ————

Prepayment requested. School/library purchase orders accepted. If not satisfied, return in 15 days for refund.

NAME _____

ADDRESS _____

_____